Atlas Collection of Acupuncture & Massage

中国针灸推拿图谱大全

Chief Editor   Zhao Xin
Translator   Li Guohua
Painter   Wang Dongsheng

Beijing Science & Technology Press
北京科学技术出版社

First Edition 1996
ISBN 7-5304-1835-1/R · 352

Atlas Collection of Acupuncture & Massage
Chief Editor   Zhao Xin
Translator   Li Guohua
Painter   Wang Dongsheng
Published by
Beijing Science & Technology Press
16 Xizhimen Nandajie, Beijing 100035, China

Distributed by
China International Book Trading Corporation
35 Chegongzhuang Xilu, Beijing 100044, China
P. O. Box 399, Beijing, China

Printed in the People's Republic of China

Preface

Acupuncture is a brilliant pearl in the treasure-house of traditional Chinese medicine and also the common wealth of the human beings. Acupuncture therapy along with massage therapy are clinically suitable for a wide range of indications. They are effective for some diseases which hardly cured by modern medicine. Acupuncture is increasingly becoming popular and accepted by the clinicians and public at home and abroad.

For the purpose of developing traditional Chinese medicine and meeting the needs of the learners of various countries, Atlas Collection of Points in Acupuncture&Massage, is now completed as a present. It is the best for those foreign friends who wants to learn acupuncture in an easy way. This atlas is also helpful to professional acupuncturists.

We believe that this atlas will bring you considerable improvement on acupuncture study.

The editor

Contents

Chapter One Standard Location of 14 Meridians' Points ·············· (1)
    Section 1 Location of Points ·············· (1)
    Section 2 Standard Location of 14 Meridians ·············· (7)
    Section 3 Location of Extra Points ·············· (68)

Chapter Two The Eight Extra Channels ·············· (75)

Chapter Three Auricular Points ·············· (81)

Chapter Four Points of Scalp Acupuncture ·············· (91)
Chapter Five Points of Hand Acupuncture ·············· (95)
Chapter Six Points of Eye Socket Acupuncture ·············· (100)
Chapter Seven Points of Nose Acupuncture ·············· (102)
Chapter Eight Points of Mouth Acupuncture ·············· (106)
Chapter Nine Points of Tongue Acupuncture ·············· (109)
Chapter Ten Points of Chest-massage Acupuncture ·············· (113)
Chapter Eleven Points of Facial Acupuncture ·············· (118)
Chapter Twolve Points of Lateral Aspect Second Metacarpal Bone Acupuncture ······ (121)
Chapter Thiteen Points of Foot Acupuncture ·············· (124)
Chapter Foureen Points of Wrist and Ankle Acupuncture ·············· (133)
Chapter Fifteen Points of Meridians and Collaterals-point Area and Belt Acupuncture ·············· (139)
Chapter Sixteen Points of Infantile Massage ·············· (144)

Chapter One
Standard Location of 14 Meridians' Points

Section 1 Location of Points

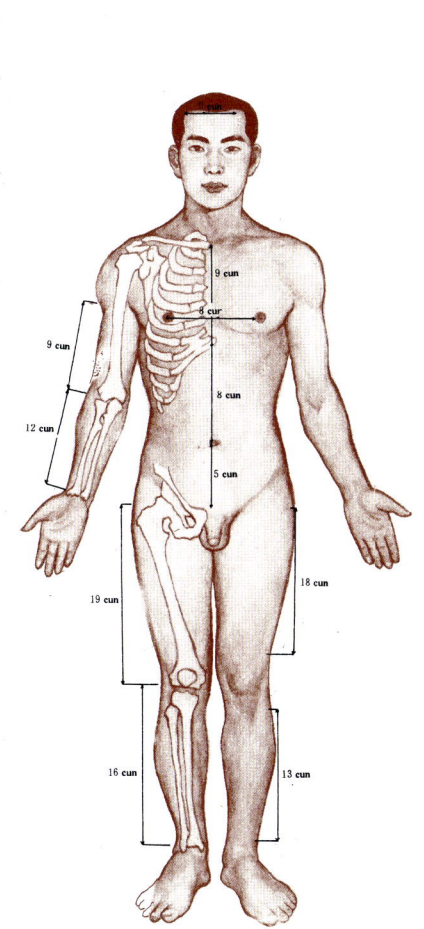
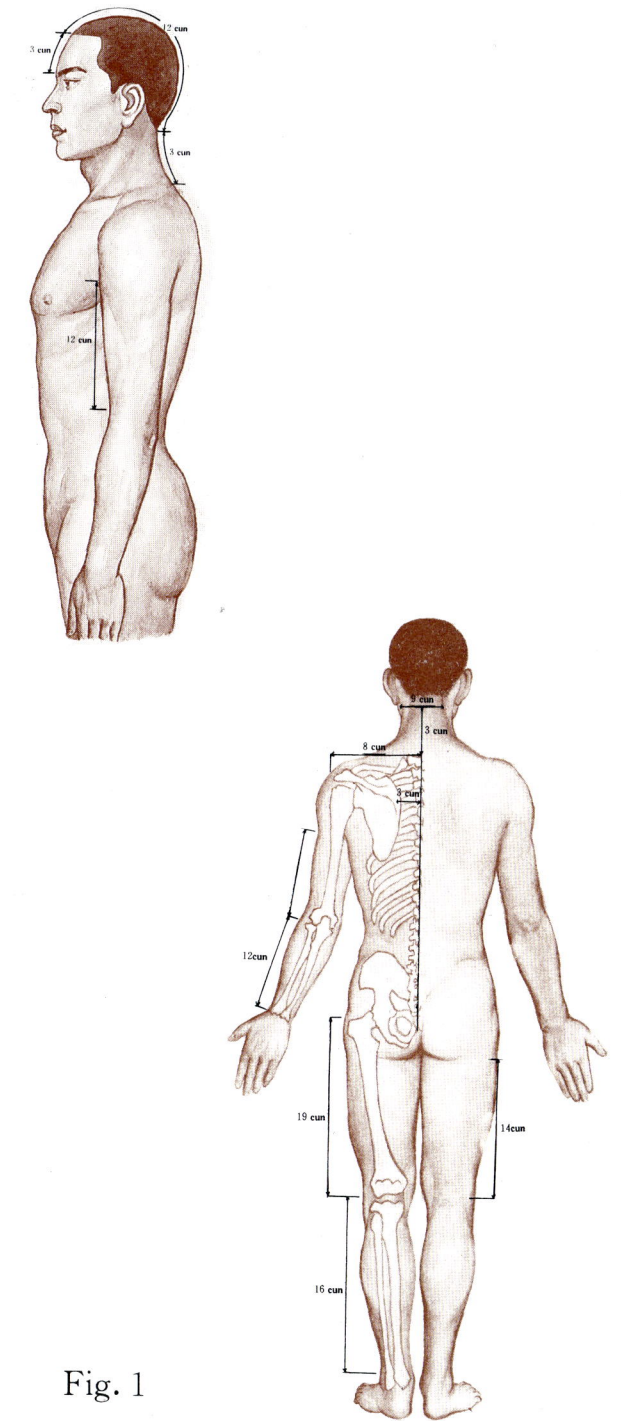

Fig. 1

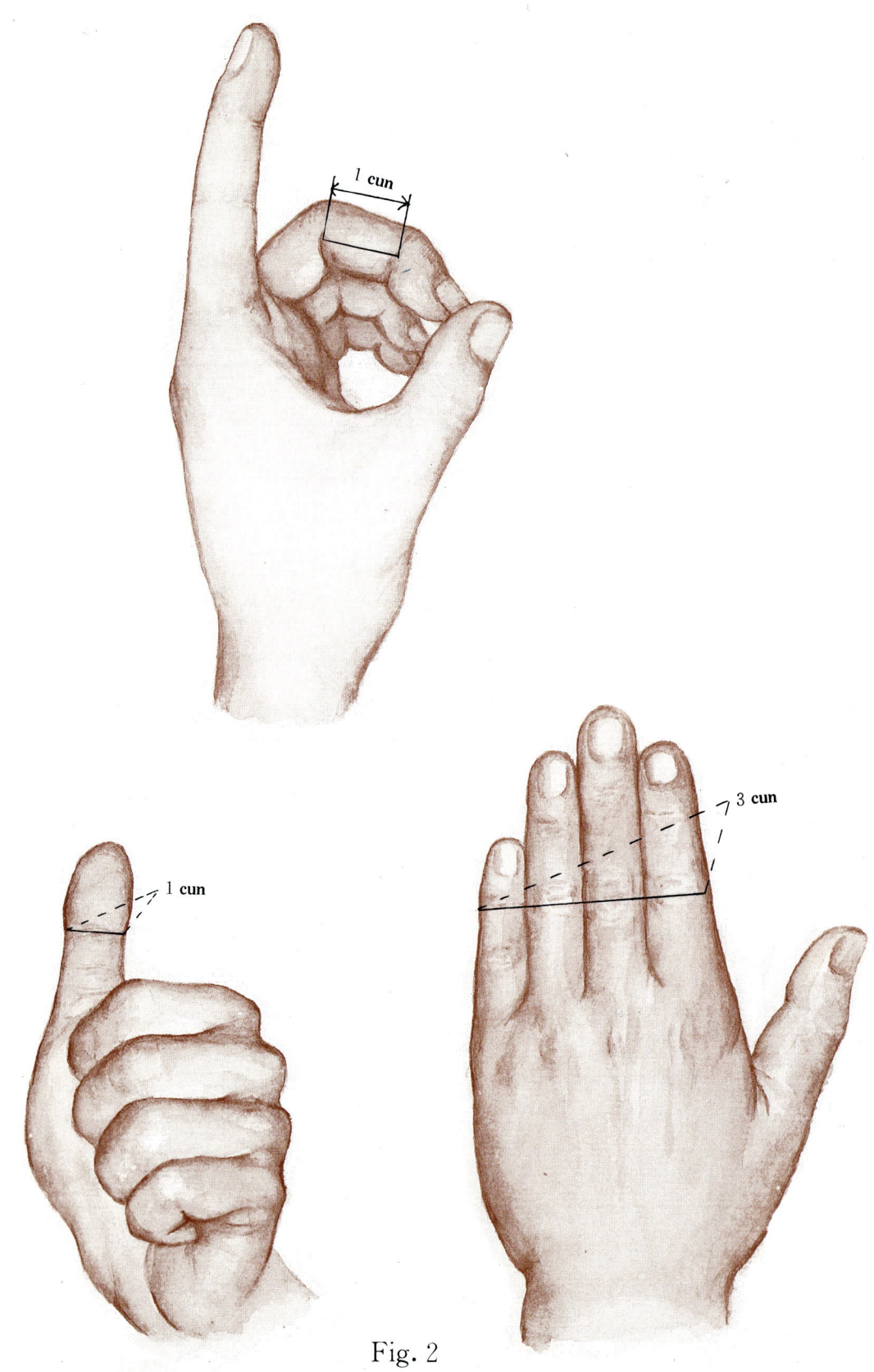

Fig. 2

There are three methods for location of points: surface anatomical landmarks, bone proportional measurement and finger measurement. They should be used in combination, but the first one is the fundamental and the other two are the supplemental ones.

1. Surface anatomical landmarks

The fixed landmarks include the prominences and depressions formed by the joints and muscles, the configuration of the five sense organs, hairline, nails and toenails. For instance, Yanglingquan(GB34) is in the depression anterior and interior to the head of fibula; Binao(LI14) is at the end of the insertion of deltoid muscle; Cuanzhu(BL2) is at the medial end of the eyebrow; Yintang(EX-HN3) is in the mid-way between the eyebrows; and Danzhong(RN17) is at the midpoint between the two nipples.

The movable landmarks refer to the clefts, depressions, wrinkles or prominences appearing on the joints, muscles, tendons and skin during motion. For example, Tinggong(SI19) is between the tragus and mandibular joint, where a depression is formed when the mouth is slightly open; Quchi(LI11) is in the depression at the lateral end of the cubital crease when the elbow is flexed.

The major anatomical landmarks on the human body surface are listed as follows:

On the head are:

the midpoint of the anterior hairline;

the midpoint of the posterior hairline;

the corner of the forehead(at the corner of the anterior hairline);

the mastoid process.

On the face are:

Yintang(EX-HN3)(at the midpoint between the eyebrow); and the pupil(in the erect sitting position and looking straight forward),or the centre of the eye(at the midpoint of the line between the inner and outer canthi).

On the neck are:

the laryngeal protuberance; and the spinous process of the 7th cervical vertebra.

On the chest are:

the suprasternal fossa(in the depression above the suprasternal notch);

the midpoint of sternoxyphoid symphysis(at the conjunction of sternum and xyphoid process); and the nipple(the center of the nipple).

On the abdomen are:

the umbilicus(Shenque, RN8)(the center of the umbilicus);

the upper border of pubic symphysis(at the crossing point of the upper border of pubic symphysis and the anterior midline); and the anterior superior iliac spine.

On the lateral side of the chest and abdomen are:

the apex of axilla(the highest point of the axillary fossa); and the free and the 11th rib.

On the back, low back and sacrum are:

the spinous process of the 7th cervical vertebra.

the spinous processes from the 1st to the 12th thoracic vertebrae and from the 1st to the 5th lumbar vertebrae.

the median sacral crest and the coccyx;

　　the medial end of the scapular spine(on the medial border of the scapula);

　　the acromial angle;

　　the posterior superior iliac spine.

　　On the upper limbs are:

　　the anterior axillary fold(the anterior end of the axillary crease);

　　the posterior axillary fold(the posterior end of the axillary crease);

　　the cubital crease;

　　the tip of elbow (olecranon),

　　the dorsal and palmar creases of wrist(the styloid crease between the distal ends of the styloid processes of ulna and radius).

　　On the lower limbs are:

　　the greater trochanter of femur;

　　the medial epicondyle of femur;

　　the medial epicondyle of tibia;

　　the inferior gluteal crease(the border between the buttocks and thigh);

　　Dubi(ST36)(in the center of the depression lateral to the patella ligament);

　　the popliteal crease;

　　the tip of the medial malleolus;

　　the tip of the lateral malleolus.

2. Bone proportional measurement

　　It is a method for location of points, in which the joints are taken as the main landmarks to measure the length and width of various portions of the human body. The proportional measurement of various portions of the human body defined in the Miraculous Pivot(Ling Shu) is taken as the basis for location of points in combination with the modified methods introduced by the acupuncturists through ages. The length between two joints is divided into several equal portions, each portion as one cun and 10 portions as one chi. The main bone proportional measurements are listed in the following table.

Table of "Bone Proportional Measurement"

Position	Origin and end points	Portion (cun)	Method of measurement	Remarks
Head and face	From the midpoint of the anterior hairline to the midpoint of the posterior hairline	12	Longitudinal measurement	Used for measuring the longitudinal distance of the points on the head
	From Yintang(EX-HN3) to the midpoint of the anterior hairline	3	Longitudinal measurement	Used for measuring the longitudinal

Region	Description	Value	Measurement Type	Usage
Head and face	Form the point below the spinous process of the 7th cervical vertebra(Dazhui. DU14) to the midpoint of the posterior hairline	3	Longitudinal measurement	
	From Yintang(EX-HN3) to the midpoint of the posterior hairline and then to the point below the spinous process of te 7th cervical vertebra(Dazhui.DU14)	18	Longitudinal measurement	
	Between the corners of forehead (Touwei. ST8)	9	Transverse measurement	Used for measuring the transverse distance of the points on the anterior part of the head
	Between the bilateral mastoid processes	9	Transverse measurement	Used for measuring the transverse distance of the points on the posterior part of the head
Chest. abdomen and hypo chon drium	From the suprasternal fossa(Tiantu. RN22) to the midpoint of the sternoxyphoid symphysis	9	Longitudinal measurement	Used for measuring the longitudinal distance of the points of the Ren Channel on the chest
	From the midpoint of the sternoxyphoid symphysis to the center of umbilicus	8	Longitudinal measurement	Used for meaasuring the longitudinal distance of the points on the upper abdomen
	From the center of the umbilicus to the upper border of the pubic symphysis(Qugu. RN2)	5	Longitudinal measurement	Used for measuring the longitudinal distance of the points on the lower abdomen
	Between the two nipples	8	Transverse measurement	Used for measuring the transverse distance of the points on the chest and abdomen
	From the apex of axilla to the free end of the 11th rib(Zhangmen. LR13)	12	Longitudinal measurement	Used for measuring the longitudinal distance of the points on the hypochondrium
Back and low back	From the medial border of the scapula to the posterior midline	3	Transverse measurement	Used for measuring the transverse distance of the points on the back
Back and low back	From the acromial angle to the posterior midline	8	Transvverse measurement	For measuring the transverse distance of the points on the shoulder and back

Upper limbs	From the anterior and posterior axillar folds to the cubital crease	9	Longitudinal measurement	Used for measuring the longitudinal distance of the points on the arm
	From the cubital crease to the dorsal crease of the wrist	12	Longitudinal measurement	Used for measuring the longitudinal distance of the points on the forearm
Low limbs	From the upper border of the pubic symphysis to the upper border of the medial epicondyle of femur	18	Longitudinal measurement	Used for measuring the longitudinal distance of the points on the three yin meridians of foot on the medial side of the lower limbs
	From the lowr border of the medial epicondyle of tibia to the tip of the medial mlleolus	13	Longitudinal measurement	Used for measuring the longitudinal poplitea crease distance of the points on the three yang meridians of foot on the latero- posterior side of the lower limbs(The distance from the gluteal groove to the popliteal crease is equivalent to 14 cun)
	From the greater trochanter to the popliteal crease	19	Longitudinal measurement	
	From the popliteal crease to the tip of the lateral malleolus	16	Longitudinal measurement	Used for measuring the longitudinal distance of the points on the three yang meridians of foot on the latero posterior side of the lower limbs

3. Finger measurement

This is a method to locate the points by measuring the distance with either the length or width of the patient's finger(s).

Middle finger measurement: When the middle finger is flexed, the distance between the radial ends of the two interphalangeal creases of the patient's middle finger is taken as 1 cun.

Thumb measurement: The width of the interphalangeal joint of the patient's thumb is taken as 1 cun.

Four-finger measurement: When the four fingers(index, middle, ring and little fingers) keep close, the width of them on the level of the proximal interphalangeal crease of the middle finger is taken as 3 cun.

This method is mainly used for locating the points of the lower limbs. When locating the points, this method should be used in combination with some simple movable landmarks on the basis of the bone proportional measurement.

Section 2
Points of 14 Meridians
1 The Lung Meridian of Hand-Taiyin

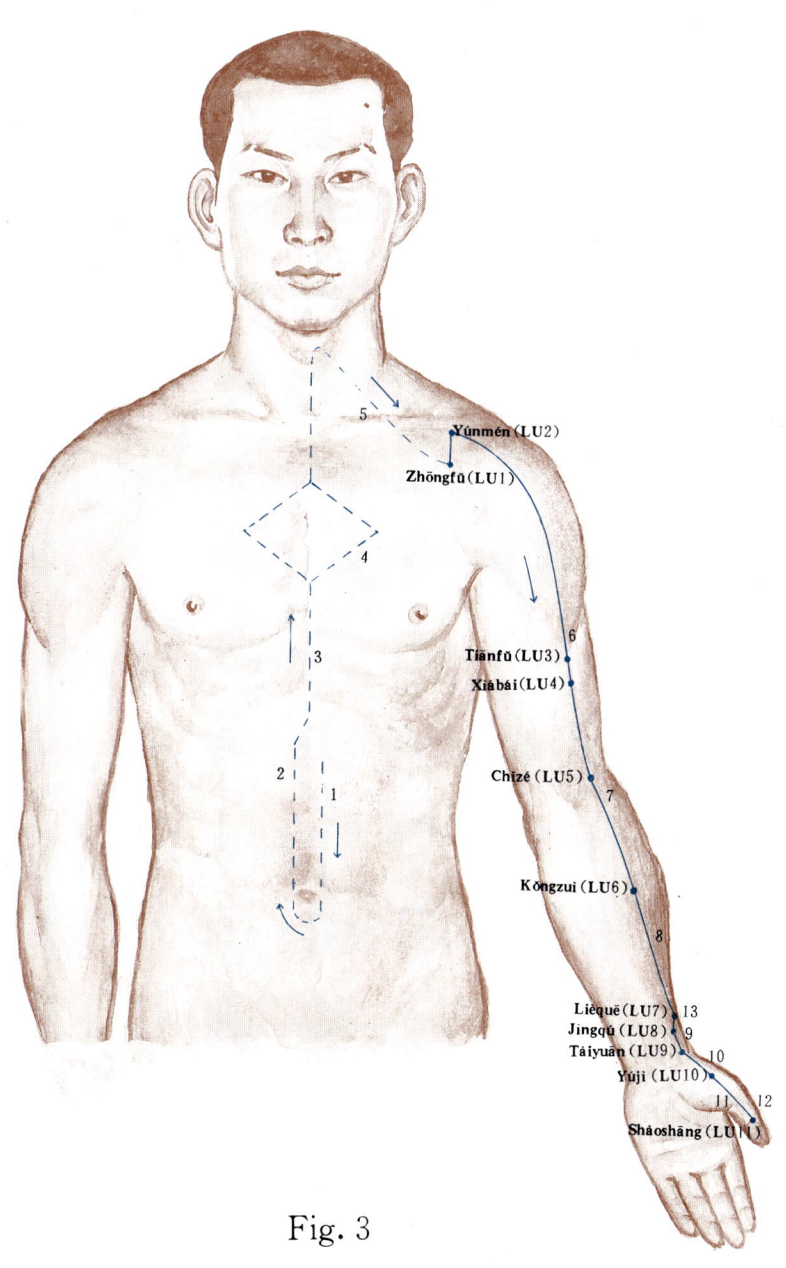

Fig. 3

(1) Course

The Lung Channel of Hand-Taiyin originates in the middle warmer, the portion between the diaphragm and the umbilicus of the body cavity, running downwards to communicate with the large intestine. Turning back, it goes along the orifices of the stomach (the pylorus and cardia), then upwards through the diaphragm into its pertaining organ, the lung. From the pulmonary series (including the trachea, throat, etc.), it comes transversely to the armpit (out of Point Zhongfu, LU1).

It then descends along the medial aspect of the upper arm, and passes in front of the Heart Channel of Hand-Shaoyin and the Pericardium Channel of Hand-Jueyin, down to the middle portion of the elbow. From there it runs along the anterior border of the radius on the medial aspect of the forearm and goes into Cunkou, the place on the wrist over the radial artery where the pulse is felt. Then it arrives at the thenar, runs along its border and emerges from the medial side of the tip of the thumb (Point Shaoshang, LU11).

The branch of the channel runs directly from the proximal aspect of the wrist (Point Lieque, LU7) into the radial side of the tip of the index (Point Shangyang, LI1), in which it connects with the Large Intestine Channel of Hand-Yangming.

(2) Points of Lung Meridian of Hand-Taiyin

Zhongfu(LU1)

Location: In the superior lateral part of the anterior thoracic wall, 1 cun below Yunmen(LU2), on the level of the 1st intercostal space, 6 cun lateral to the anterior midline.

Indication: cough with dyspnea, stuffiness in the chest and pain in the chest, shoulder or back.

Yunmen(LU2)

Location: In the superior lateral part of the anterior thoracic wall, superior to the coracoid process of scapula, in the depression of the infraclavicular fossa, 6 cun lateral to the anterior midline.

Indications: Cough with dyspnea, irritable and distending sensation in the chest, chest pain, pain in the shoulder and arm.

Tianfu(LU3)

Location: On the medial side of the upper arm and on the radial border of biceps.

Indications: Dyspnea, epistaxis, pain in the medial portion of the upper arm.

Xiabai(LU4)

Location: On the medial side of the upper arm and on the radial border of biceps muscle of arm, 4 cun below the anterior end of the axillary fold, or 5cun above the cubital crease.

Indications: Cough, irritable and distending sensation in the chest, pain in the medial portion of the upper arm.

Chize(LU5)

Location: In the cubital crease, in the depression of the radial side of the tendon of biceps muscle of arm.

Indications: Cough, hemoptysis, hectic fever, dyspnea, sore-throat, distention in the chest, infantile convulsion, contraction of the elbow and arm, pain in the breast.

Kongzui(LU6)

Location: On the radial side of the palmar surface of the forearm, and on the line connecting Chize(LU5) and Taiyuan(LU9), 7 cun above the cubital crease.

Indications: Cough with dyspnea, chest pain, hemoptysis, sore-throat, contraction of the elbow and arm.

Lieque(LU7)

Location: On the radial side of the forearm, proximal to the styloid process of radius, 1.5 cun above the crease of the wrist, between brachioradial muscle and the tendon of long abductor muscle of the thumb.

Indications: Headache, stiffness of the nape, cough with dyspnea, sore-throat, hemiparalysis of face, toothache, weakness and pain in the wrist.

Jingqu(LU8)

Location: On the radial side of the palmar surface of the forearm, one cun above the crease of the wrist, in the depression between styloid process of radius and radial artery.

Indications: Cough with dyspnea, fever, chest pain, sore-throat, pain in the wrist.

Taiyuan(LU9)

Location: At the radial end of the crease of the wrist, where the pulsation of radial artery is palpable.

Indications: Cough with dyspnea, hemoptysis, sore-throat, chest pain, palpitation, pain in the arm and wrist.

Yuji(LU10)

Location: In the depression proximal to the 1st metacarpophalangeal joint, on the radial side of the midpoint of the metacarpal bone, and on the junction of the red and white skin.

Indications: Cough, hemoptysis, sore-throat, aphonia, fever, feverish sensation in the palms.

Shaoshang(LU11)

Location: On the radial side of the distal segment of the thumb, 0.1 cun from the corner of the nail.

Indications: Sore-throat, cough with dyspnea, epistaxis, fever, coma, manic-depressive psychosis, contraction of the thumb.

2. The Large Intestine Meridian of Hand-Yangming

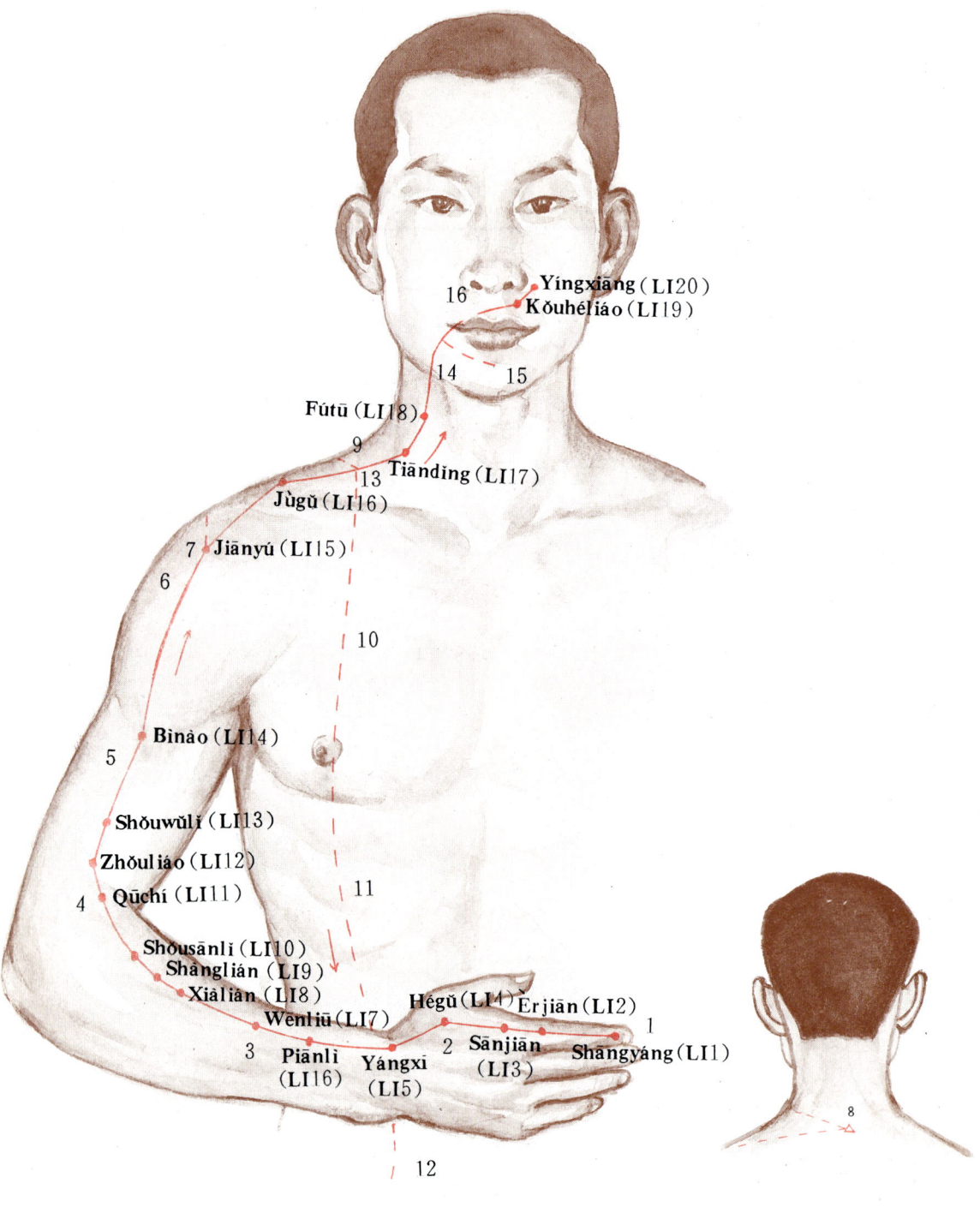

Fig. 4

(1) Course

This channel starts from the tip of the radial side of the index (Point Shangyang, LI1). It runs upwards along the radial side of the index and passes between the ossa metacarpalia I and II, goes into the depression between the tendons of m. extensor pollicis longus and brevis, then along the antero-lateral aspect of the forearm to the lateral side of the elbow (Point Quchi, LI11). Along the anterior border of the lateral side of the upper arm, it ascends to the highest point of the shoulder (Point Jianyu, LI15), and then goes along the anterior border of the acromion up to 7th cervical vertebra (Point Dazhui, DU14), from where it comes downwards into the supraclavicular fossa and communicates with the lung. Descending through the diaphragm, it enters its pertaining organ, the large intestine.

The branch channel from the supraclavicular fossa runs upwards to the neck, passes through the cheek, and enters into the lower teeth and gum. Then it curves round the lips and meets at Point Renzhong(DU26), or philtrum, thevertical groove on the mid-line of the upper lip. From there the channel ofthe left side turns right, while the right side channel turns left. They go upwards to both sides of the wings of the nose (Point Yingxiang, LI20) and connect with the Stomach Channel of Foot-Yangming.

(2) Points of Large Intestine Meridian of Hand-Yangming

Shangyang(LI1)

Location: On the radial side of the distal segment of the index finger, 0.1cun from the corner of the nail.

Indications: Toothache, sore-throat, submental swelling, numbness of the fingers, fever with no perspiration, coma.

Erjian(LI2)

Location: In the depression of the radial side, distal to the 2nd metacarpophalangeal joint when a loose fist is made.

Indications: Blurred vision, epistaxis, toothache, sore-throat, fever.

Sanjian(LI3)

Location: In the depression of the radial side, proximal to the 2nd metacarpal bones, and on the radial side of the midpoint of the 2nd metacarpal bone.

Indications: Ophthalmalgia, toothache, sore-throat, inflammation of the fingers and the back of the hand.

Hegu(LI4)

Location: On the dorsum of the hand, between the 1st and 2nd metacarpal bones, and on the radial side of the midpoint of the 2nd metacarpal bone.

Indications: Headache, pain in the neck and nape, conjunctival congestion and swelling pain in the eye, epistaxis, stuffy nose, rhinorrhea with turbid discharge, toothache, deafness, edema of face, sore-throat, mumps, lockjaw, facial hemiparalysis, fever with either anhidrosis or hyperhidrosis, abdominal pain, dysentery, constipation, brachialgia in the upper arm, flaccidity, infantile convulsion, amenorrhea, dystocia.

Yangxi(LI5)

Location: At the radial end of the crease of the wrist, in the depression between the tendons of short extensor and long extensor muscles of the thumb when the thumb is upward tilted.

Indications: Headache, conjunctival congestion and swelling pain in the eye, toothache, sore-throat, pain in the wrist.

Pianli(LI6)

Location: With the elbow slightly flexed, on the radial side of the dorsal surface of the forearm, and on the line connecting Yangxi(LI5) and Quchi(LI11), 3 cun above the crease of the wrist.

Indications: conjunctival congestion, tinnitus, deafness, nasal bleeding, brachialgia, sore-throat, edema.

Wenliu(LI7)

Location: With the elbow flexed, on the radial side of the dorsal surface of the forearm and on the line connecting Yangxi(LI5) and Quchi(LI11), 5 cun above the crease of the wrist.

Indications: Headache, edema of face, sore-throat, borborygmus, abdominal pain, aching pain in the elbow and arm.

Xialian(LI8)

Location: On the radial side of the dorsal surface of the forearm and on the line connecting Yangxi(LI5) and Quchi(LI11), 4 cun below the cubital crease.

Indications: Abdominal pain, borborygmus, brachialgia, paralysis of the arm.

Shanglian(LI9)

Location: On the radial side of the dorsal surface of the forearm and on the line connecting Yangxi(LI5) and Quchi(LI11), 3 cun below the cubital crease.

Indications: Aching pain in the shoulder and arm, paralysis and numbness of the arm, borborygmus, abdominal pain.

Shousanli(LI10)

Location: On the radial side of the dorsal surface of the forearm and on the line connecting Yangxi(LI5) and Quchi(LI11), 2 cun below the cubital crease.

Indications: Abdominal pain, diarrhea, toothache, submental swelling, paralysis of the arm, pain in the back and shoulder.

Quchi(LI11)

Location: With the elbow flexed, at the lateral end of the cubital crease, at the midpoint of the line connecting Chize(LU5) and external humeral epicondyle.

Indications: Sore-throat, toothache, conjunctival congestion and ophthalmalgia, rubella, scrofula, paralysis of the arm, abdominal pain accompanied with vomiting and diarrhea, fever.

Zhouliao(LI12)

Location: With the elbow flexed, on the lateral side of the upper arm, 1 cun above Quchi(LI11), on the border of humerus.

Indications: Aching pain and numbness or contraction of the elbow and arm.

Shouwuli(LI13)

Location: On the lateral side of the upper arm and on the line connecting Quchi(LI11) and Jianyu(LI15), 3 cun above Quchi(LI11).

Indications: Contraction of the elbow and arm, brachialgia, scrofula.

Binao(LI14)

Location: On the lateral side of the arm, at the insertion of deltoid muscle and on the line connecting Quchi(LI11) and Jianyu(LI15), 7 cun above Quchi(LI11).

Indications: Pain in the shoulder and arm, paralysis of the arm, stiffness of the neck and nape, scrofula.

Jianyu(LI15)

Location: On the shoulder, superior to the deltoid muscle, in the depression anterior and inferior to acromion when the arm is abducted or raised on the level of the shoulder.

Indications: Pain in the shoulder and arm, paralysis of the arm, rubella, scrofula.

Jugu(LI16)

Location: On the shoulder, in the depression between the acromial extremity of the clavicle and scapular spine.

Indications: Inability to raise arm due to pain in the shoulder and arm, backache.

Tianding(LI17)

Location: On the lateral side of the neck, at the posterior border of sternocleidomastoid muscle beside the laryngeal protuberance, at the midpoint of the line connecting Futu(LI18) and Quepen(ST12).

Indications: Sudden loss of voice, sore-throat, scrofula, goiter due to Qi disorders.

Futu(LI18)

Location: On the lateral side of the neck, beside the laryngeal protuberance, between the anterior and posterior borders of sternocleidomastoid muscle.

Indications: Cough with dyspnea, sore-throat, sudden loss of voice, scrofula, goiter due to Qi disorders.

Kouheliao(LI19)

Location: On the upper lip, directly below the lateral border of the nostril, on the level of Shuigou(DU26).

Indications: Stuffy nose, nasal bleeding, facial hemiparalysis.

Yingxiang(LI20)

Location: In the nasolabial groove, beside the midpoint of the lateral border of nasal ala.

Indications: Stuffy nose, anosmia, rhinorrhea with turbid discharge, facial hemiparalysis, itching or edema of the face.

3. The Stomach Channel of Foot-Yangming

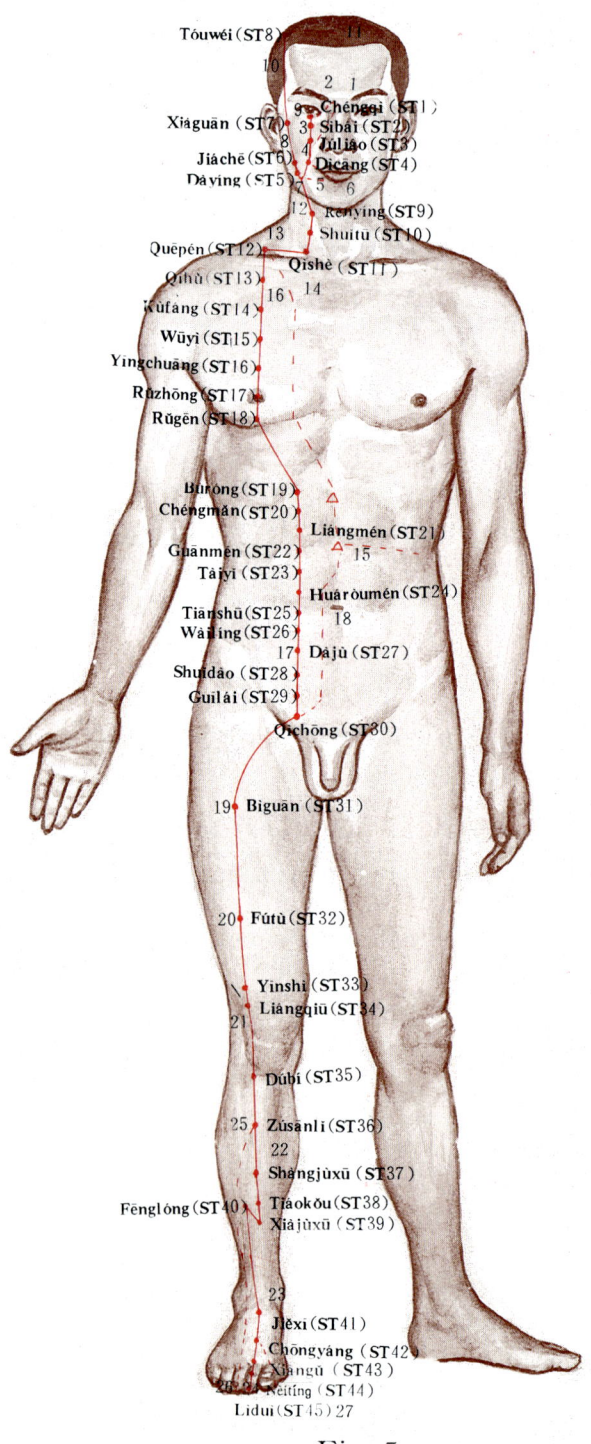

Fig. 5

(1) Course

This channel starts from the side of the nose (Point Yingxiang, LI20), and ascends to the root of the nose, meeting the Urinary Bladder Channel (at Point Jingming, BL1). Then it descends along the lateral side of the nose and enters into the upper gum. Emerging and curving round the lips, it passes downwards and connects with the symmetrical channel at Point Chengjiang(RN24) in the sulcus mentolabiabialis. And it runs along the posterior-inferior side of the parotid gland, through Point Daying(ST5), and Point Jiache(ST6) in succession, and then ascends in front of the ear, through Point Shangguan(GB3), the point of the Gall Bladder Channel of Foot-Shaoyang. And finally, it runs along the hairline and reaches the forehead (Point Touwei, ST8).

One of its branches sprouts in front of Daying(ST5), descends to Renying(ST9), and goes along the throat into the supraclavicular fossa. From there it descends through the diaphragm, enters into its pertaining organ, the stomach, and communicates with the spleen.

A straight branch from the supraclavicular fossa descends to the medial border of the papilla mammae. Then it makes its descent along the side of the umbilicus and enters into Point Qichong(ST30).

One of the branches starting from the pylorus descends through the abdominal cavity, and joins the straight branch at Point Qichong(ST30). From there it descends through Point Biguan(ST31), Futu(ST35), to the knee. Along the anterolateral aspect of the tibia, it goes towards the dorsum of the foot, and then to the lateral side of the tip of the second toe (Point Lidui, ST45).

Another branch sprouting from the region 3 individual cun below the genu(Point Zusanli, ST36), descends to the lateral side of the middle toe.

The branch sprouting from the dorsum of the foot (Point Chongyang, ST42)descends into the medial margin of the hallux, and through its tip (Point Yinbai, SP1), connects with the Spleen Channel of Foot-Taiyin.

(2) Points of the Stomach Meridian of Foot-Yangming, ST

Chengqi(ST1)

Location: On the face, directly below the pupil, between the eyeball and the infraorbital ridge.

Indications: Conjunctival congestion, epiphora, night blindness, twitching of eyelid, facial hemiparalysis.

Push the eyeball upward slightly with the left thumb and puncture perpendicularly 0.3-0.7 cun along the infraorbital ridge. It is not advisable to manipulate theneedle with large amplitude, to spare the blood vessel from hematoma.

Sibai(ST2)

Location: On the face, directly below the pupil, in the depression of the infraorbital foramen.

Indications: conjunctival congestion, ophthalmalgia, itching of eyes, facial paralysis, twitching of eyelid, prosopodynia.

Juliao(ST3)

Location: On the face, directly below the pupil, on the level of the lower border of the nasal ala, beside the nasolabial groove.

Indications: Facial paralysis, twitching of eyelid, epistaxis, toothache, swelling of the lips and cheek.

Dicang(ST4)

Location: On the face, directly below the pupil, beside the mouth angle.

Indications: Facial paralysis, salivation, twitching of eyelid.

Daying(ST5)

Location: Anterior to the mandibular angle, on the anterior border of the masseter muscle, where the pulsation of the facial artery is palpable.

Indications: Facial paralysis, lockjaw, edema of cheek, prosopodynia, toothache.

Jiache(ST6)

Location: On the cheek, one finger breadth (middle finger) anterior and superior to the mandibular angle, in the depression where the masseter muscle is prominent.

Indications: Facial hemiparalysis, toothache, buccal swelling, edema of face, mumps, lockjaw.

Xiaguan(ST7)

Location: On the face, anterior to the ear, in the depression between the zygomatic arch and mandibular notch.

Indications: Deafness, tinnitus, toothache, facial paralysis, prosopodynia, dyscinesia of maxillary joint.

Touwei(ST8)

Location: On the lateral side of the head, 0.5 cun above the anterior hairline at the corner of the forehead, and 4.5 cun lateral to the midline of the head.

Indications: Headache, vertigo, ophthalmalgia, epiphora.

Renying(ST9)

Location: On the neck, beside the laryngeal protuberance, and on the anterior border of the sternocleidomastoid muscle where the pulsation of the common carotid artery is palpable.

Indications: Sore-throat, dyspnea, goiter due to Qi disorders, dizziness, flushed face.

Shuitu(ST10)

Location: On the neck and on the anterior border of the sternocleidomastoid muscle, at the midpoint of the line connecting Renying(ST9) and Qishe(ST11)

Indications: Sore-throat, dyspnea, cough.

Qishe(ST11)

Location: On the neck and on the upper border of the medial end of the clavicle, between the sternal and clavicular heads of the sternocleidomastoid muscle.

Indications: Sore throat, stiffness of the nape, dyspnea, hiccup, goiter.

Quepen(ST12)

Location: At the centre of the supraclavicular fossa, 4 cun lateral to the anterior midline.

Indication: Cough with dyspnea, sore-throat, pain in the supraclavicular fossa.

Qihu(ST13)

Location: On the chest, below the midpoint of the lower border of the clavicle, 4 cun lateral to the anterior midline.

Indications: Fullness sensation in the chest, cough with dyspnea, hiccup, pain in the chest and hypochondriac region.

Kufang(ST14)

Location: On the chest, in the 2nd intercostal space, 4 cun lateral to the anterior midline.

Indications: Distending pain in the chest and hypochondriac region, cough.

Wuyi(ST15)

Location: On the chest, in the 2nd intercostal space, 4 cun lateral to the anterior midline.

Indications: Distending pain in the chest and hypochondriac region, cough with dyspnea, mastitis.

Yingchuang(ST16)

Location: On the chest, in the 3rd intercostal space, 4 cun lateral to the anterior midline.

Indications: Distending pain in the chest and hypochondriac region, cough with dyspnea, mastitis.

Ruzhong(ST17)
Location: On the chest, in the 4th intercostal space, at the centre of the nipple, 4 cun lateral to the anterior midline.

Method: Acupuncture and moxibustion prohibited. Used for measuring the transverse distance of the points on the chest and abdomen. The distance between the two nipples is taken as 8 cun.

Rugen(ST18)
Location: On the chest, directly below the nipple, on the lower border of the breast, in the 5th intercostal space, 4 cun lateral to the anterior midline.

Indications: chest pain, cough with dyspnea, mastitis, lack of lactation.

Burong(ST19)
Location: On the upper abdomen, 6 cun above the centre of the umbilicus and 2 cun lateral to the anterior midline.

Indications: Distention of the abdomen, vomiting, stomachache, loss of appetite.

Chengman(ST20)
Location: On the upper abdomen, 5 cun above the centre of the umbilicus and 2 cun lateral to the anterior midline.

Indications: Distention of the abdomen, vomiting, stomachache, loss of appetite.

Liangmen(ST21)
Location: On the upper abdomen, r cun above the centre of the umbilicus and 2 cun lateral to the anterior midline.

Indications: Distention of the abdomen, vomiting, stomachache, loss of appetite, diarrhea.

Guanmen(ST22)
Location: On the upper abdomen, 3 cun above the centre of the umbilicus and 2 cun lateral to the anterior midline.

Indications: Distention and pain in the abdomen, poor appetite, diarrhea, borborygmus, edema.

Taiyi(ST23)
Location: On the upper abdomen, 2 cun above the centre of the umbilicus and 2 cun lateral to the anterior midline.

Indications: Stomachache, irritability, manic-depressive psychosis, indigestion.

Huaroumen(ST24)
Location: On the upper abdomen, 1 cun above the centre of the umbilicus and 2 cun lateral to the anterior midline.

Indications: Stomachache, vomiting, manic-depressive psychosis.

Tianshu(ST25)
Location: On the middle abdomen, 2 cun lateral to the centre of the umbilicus.

Indications: Abdominal distension, borborygmus, pain around the umbilicus, constipation, diarrhea, abdominal mass, dysentery, irregular menstruation.

Wailing(ST26)
Location: On the lower abdomen, 1 cun below the centre of the umbilicus and 2 cun lateral to the anterior midline.

Indications: Abdominal pain, hernia, dysmenorrhea.

Daju(ST27)
Location: On the lower abdomen, 2 cun below the centre of the umbilicus and 2 cun lateral to the anterior mid-

line.

Indications: Distention of the lower abdomen, dribbling urination, hernia, emission, premature ejaculation.

Shuidao(ST28)

Location: On the lower abdomen, 3 cun below the centre of the umbilicus and 2cun lateral to the anterior midline

Indications: Distention of the lower abdomen, anuresis, edema, hernia, dysmenorrhea, sterility.

Guilai(ST29)

Location: On the lower abdomen, 4 cun below the centre of the umbilicus and 2 cun lateral to the anterior midline.

Indications: Abdominal pain, hernia, irregular menstruation, leukorrhagia, spermatorrhea, impotence, prolapse of the uterus.

Qichong(ST30)

Location: Slightly above the inguinal groove, 5 cun below the centre of the umbilicus and 2 cun lateral to the anterior midline.

Indications: Abdominal pain with borborygmus, hernia, swelling pain in vulva, impotence, dysmenorrhea, irregular menstruation.

Biguan(ST31)

Location: On the anterior side of the thigh and on the line connecting the anteriosuperior iliac spine and the superiolateral corner of the patella, on the level of the perineum when the thigh is flexed, in the depression lateral to the sartorius muscle.

Indications: Flaccidity of lower limbs, pain in thigh and dyskinesia of the lower extremities.

Futu(ST32)

Location: On the anterior side of the thigh and on the line connecting the anteriosuperior iliac spine and the superiolateral corner of the patella, 3cun above this corner.

Indications: Pain in the lumbar region, hernia, beriberi, paralysis and pain of the lower extremities.

Yinshi(ST33)

Location: On the anterior side of the thigh and on the line connecting anteriosuperior iliac spine and the superiolateral corner of the patella, 3 cun above this corner.

Indications: Numbness and aching pain in the leg especially the knee, dyskinesia or paralysis of the lower extremities.

Liangqiu(ST34)

Location: With the knee flexed, on the anterior side of the thigh and on the line connecting the anterosuperior iliac spine and the superolateral corner of the patella, 2 cun above this corner.

Indications: Pain and numbness of the knee and leg, gastric pain, breast abscess, paralysis of the lower extremities.

Dubi(ST35)

Location: With the knee flexed, on the knee, in the depression lateral to the patella and its ligament.

Indications: Gonalgia, numbness and dyskinesia of knee, flaccidity of lowerlimbs.

Zusanli(ST36)

Location: On the anterior lateral side of the leg, 3 cun below Dubi(ST35), one finger breadth(middle finger) from the anterior crest of the tibia.

Indications: Gastric pain, abdominal distension, vomiting, diarrhea, dysentery, emaciation due to general deficiency, constipation, acute appendicitis, numbness and pain of the lower extremities, edema, manic-depressive psychosis.

Shangjuxu(ST37)

Location: On the anterolateral side of the leg, 6 cun below Dubi(ST35), one finger breadth (middle finger) from the anterior crest of the tibia.

Indications: Borborygmus, abdominal pain, diarrhea, constipation, acute appendicitis, muscular atrophy, numbness, pain and flaccidity of the lower extremities.

Tiaokou(ST38)

Location: On the anterolateral side of the leg, 9 cun below Dubi(ST35), one finger breadth (middle finger) from the anterior crest of the tibia.

Indications: Numbness and aching pain in the leg, flaccidity of foot, inability to raise arm due to pain in the shoulder and arm, epigastric pain.

Xiajuxu(ST39)

Location: On the anterolateral side of the leg, 9 cun below Dubi(ST35), one finger breadth (middle finger) from the anterior crest of the tibia.

Indications: Pain in the lower abdomen, lumbago radiating to the testes, pain in the breast, flaccidity of the lower limbs.

Fenglong(ST40)

Location: On the anterolateral side of the leg, 8 cun above the tip of the external malleolus, lateral to Tiaokou (ST38), and two finger breadths (middle finger) from the anterior crest of the tibia.

Indications: Headache and dizziness, cough with dyspnea, abundant expectoration, chest pain, constipation, manic-depressive psychosis, epilepsy, swelling pain or flaccidity of lower limbs.

Jiexi(ST41)

Location: In the central depression of the crease between the instep of the foot and leg, between the tendons of the long extensor muscle of the great toe and the long extensor muscle of the toes.

Indications: Pain in ankle joint, flaccidity of lower limbs, depressive psychosis, headache, dizziness, distention of the abdomen, constipation.

Chongyang(ST42)

Location: On the dome of the instep of the foot, between the tendons of the long extensor muscle of the great toe and the long extensor muscle of the toes, where the pulsation of the dorsal artery of the foot is palpable.

Indications: Toothache, red swelling of the dorsum pedis, facial hemiparalysis, weakness of foot.

Xiangu(ST43)

Location: On the instep of the foot, in the depression distal to the commissure of the 2nd and 3rd metatarsal bones.

Indications: Edema, abdominal pain, borborygmus, swelling pain in the dorsum pedis.

Neiting(ST44)

Location: On the instep of the foot, at the junction of the red and white skin proximal to the margin of the web between the 2nd and 3rd toes.

Indications: Toothache, prosopodynia, facial hemiparalysis, sore-throat, nasal bleeding, stomachache, acid regurgitation, distention of abdomen, diarrhea, dysentery, constipation, swelling pain in the dorsum pedis, fever.

Lidui(ST45)

Location: On the lateral side of the distal segment of the 2nd toe, 0.1 cun from the corner of the toenail.

Indications: Edema of face, epistaxis, facial hemiparalysis, toothache, inflammation of the throat, abdominal distention, cold legs and feet, fever, dreaminess, manic-depressive psychosis.

4. The Spleen Meridian of Foot-Taiyin

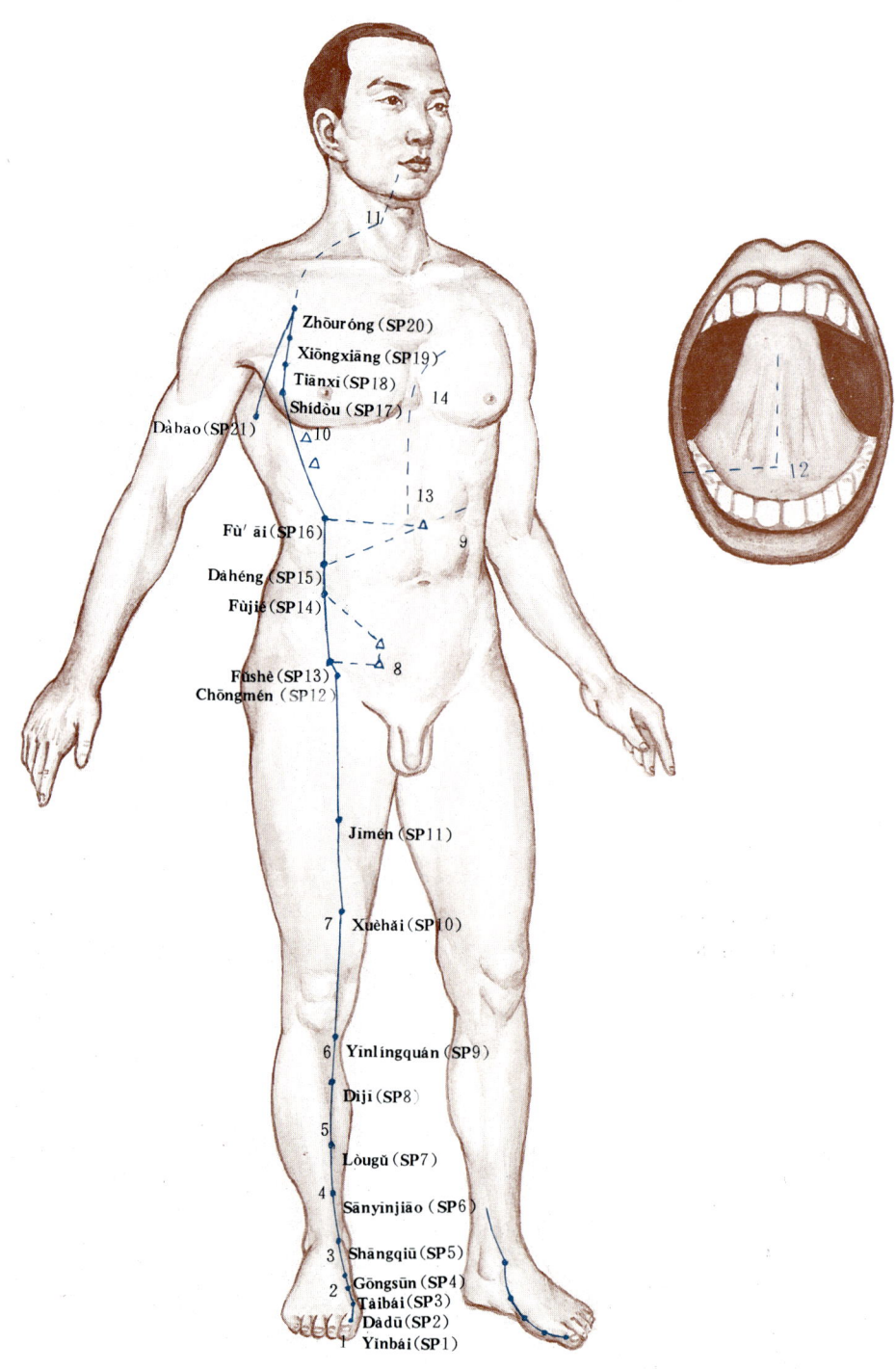

Fig. 6

(1) Course

The channel starts from the tip of the medial side of the great toe (Yin-bai, SP1). From there it runs along the junction of the red and white skin of the medial aspect of the great toe, passes the posterior surface of "Hegu", the nodular process on the medial aspect of the first metatarsophalangeal joint and ascends in front of the medial malleolus to the medial aspect of the calf. It makes its way along the posterior border of the tibia, ascends in front of the Liver Channel of Foot-Jueyin, goes through the anterior medial aspect of the knee and thigh, and into the abdominal cavity, then enters its pertaining organ, the spleen, and communicates with the stomach. From there it goes through the diaphragm, and upwards along the two sides of the throat, reaches the root of the tongue and spreads over its lower surface.

The branch of the channel sprouts from the stomach, goes upwards through the diaphragm, disperse into the heart and connects with Heart Channel of Hand-Shaoyin.

(2) Points of the Spleen Meridian of Foot-Taiyin, SP

Yinbai(SP1)

Location: On the medial side of the distal segment of the great toe, 0.1 cun from the corner of the toenail.

Indications: Abdominal distention, hematochezia, menorrhagia, metrorrhagia and metrostaxis, manic-depressive psychosis, dreaminess, infantile convulsion.

Dadu(SP2)

Location: On the medial border of the foot, in the depression of the junction of the red and white skin, anterior and inferior to the 1st metatarsophalangeal joint.

Indications: Abdominal distention, stomachache, constipation, fever with anhidrosis.

Taibai(SP3)

Location: On the medial border of the foot, in the depression of the junction of the red and white skin, posterior and inferior to the 1st metatarsophalangeal joint.

Indications: Stomachache, abdominal distention, constipation, dysentery, vomiting and diarrhea, borborygmus, heavy sensation of the body, beriberi.

Gongsun(SP4)

Location: On the medial border of the foot, anterior and inferior to the proximal end of the 1st metatarsal bone.

Indications: Stomachache, vomiting, abdominal pain, distention of the abdomen, diarrhea, dysentery, borborygmus.

Shangqiu(SP5)

Location: In the depression anterior and inferior to the medial malleolus, at the midpoint of the line connecting the tuberosity of the navicular bone and the tip of the medial malleolus.

Indications: Distention of the abdomen, constipation, diarrhea, borborygmus, glossalgia and stiff tongue, pain in the ankle, hemorrhoid.

Sanyinjiao(SP6)

Location: On the medial side of the leg, 3 cun above the tip of the medial malleolus, posterior to the medial border of the tibia.

Indications: Abdominal pain, borborygmus, distention of the abdomen, diarrhea, dysmenorrhea, irregular menstruation, metrostaxis and metrorrhagia, abnormal vaginal discharge, prolapse of uterus, infertility, dystocia, emission, impotency, enuresis, dysuria, edema, hernia, pain in the vulva, flaccidity of the lower extremities, headache, dizziness, insomnia.

Lougu(SP7)

Location: On the medial side of the leg and on the line connecting the tip of the medial malleolus and Yinlingquan (SP9), 6 cun from the tip of the medial malleolus, posterior to the medial border of the tibia.

Indications: Distention of the abdomen, borborygmus, coldness and numbness of the lower limbs.

Diji(SP8)

Location: On the medial side of the leg and on the line connecting the tip of the medial malleolus and Yinlingquan (SP9), 6 cun from the tip of the medial malleolus, posterior to the medial border of the tibia.

Indications: Abdominal pain, distention of the abdomen, diarrhea, edema, dysuria, emission, irregular menstruation, dysmenorrhea.

Yinlingquan(SP9)

Location: On the medial side of the leg, in the depression posterior and inferior to the medial condyle of the tibia.

Indications: Abdominal pain, distention in the abdomen, diarrhea, dysentery, edema, jaundice, dysuria, enuresis, urinary incontinence, pain in the vulva, dysmenorrhea, gonalgia.

Xuehai(SP10)

Location: With the knee flexed, on the medial side of the thigh, 2 cun above the superior medial corner of the patella, on the prominence of the medial head of the quadriceps muscle of the thigh.

Indications: Irregular menstruation, dysmenorrhea, metrorrhagia or metrostaxis, amenorrhea, rubella, eczema, erysipelas, pain in the medial part of the thigh.

Jimen(SP11)

Location: On the medial side of the thigh and on the line connecting Xuehai(SP10) and Chongmen(SP12), 6 cun above Xuehai(SP10).

Indications: Bradyuria, enuresis, swelling pain in the inguinal region, flaccidity of the lower limbs.

Chongmen(SP12)

Location: At the lateral end of the inguinal groove, 3.5 cun lateral to the midpoint of the upper border of the symphysis pubis, lateral to the pulsating external iliac artery.

Indications: Abdominal pain, hernia, bradyuria.

Fushe(SP13)

Location: On the lower abdomen, 4 cun below the centre of the umbilicus, 0.7 cun above Chongmen(SP12), and 4 cun lateral to the anterior midline.

Indications: Pain in the lower abdomen, hernia.

Fujie(SP14)

Location: On the lower abdomen, 1.3 cun below Daheng(SP15), and 4 cun lateral to the anterior midline.

Indications: Pain around the umbilicus, abdominal distention, hernia, diarrhea, constipation.

Daheng(SP15)

Location: On the middle abdomen, 4 cun lateral to the centre of the umbilicus.

Indications: Abdominal pain and distention, diarrhea, dysentery, constipation.

Fu'ai(SP16)

Location: On the upper abdomen, 3 cun above the centre of the umbilicus, and 4 cun lateral to the anterior midline.

Indications: Pain in the abdomen, indigestion, constipation, dysentery.

Shidou(SP17)

Location: On the lateral side of the chest and in the 5th intercostal space, 6 cun lateral to the anterior midline.
Indications: Distending pain in the chest and hypochondriac region.

Tianxi(SP18)

Location: On the lateral side of the chest and in the 4th intercostal space, 6 cun lateral to the anterior midline.
Indications: Distending pain in the chest and hypochondriac region, cough, dyspnea, mastitis, lack of lactation.

Xiongxiang(SP19)

Location: On the lateral side of the chest and in the 3rd intercostal space, 6 cun lateral to the anterior midline.
Indications: Distending pain in the chest and hypochondriac region.

Zhourong(SP20)

Location: On the lateral side of the chest and in the 2nd intercostal space, 6 cun lateral to the anterior midline.
Indications: Distention in the chest and hypochondriac region, cough with dyspnea.

Dabao(SP21)

Location: On the lateral side of the chest and on the middle axillary line, in the 6th intercostal space.
Indications: Pain in the chest and hypochondriac region, dyspnea, pantalgia, lassitude of the extremities.

5. The Heart Meridian of Hand-Shaoyin

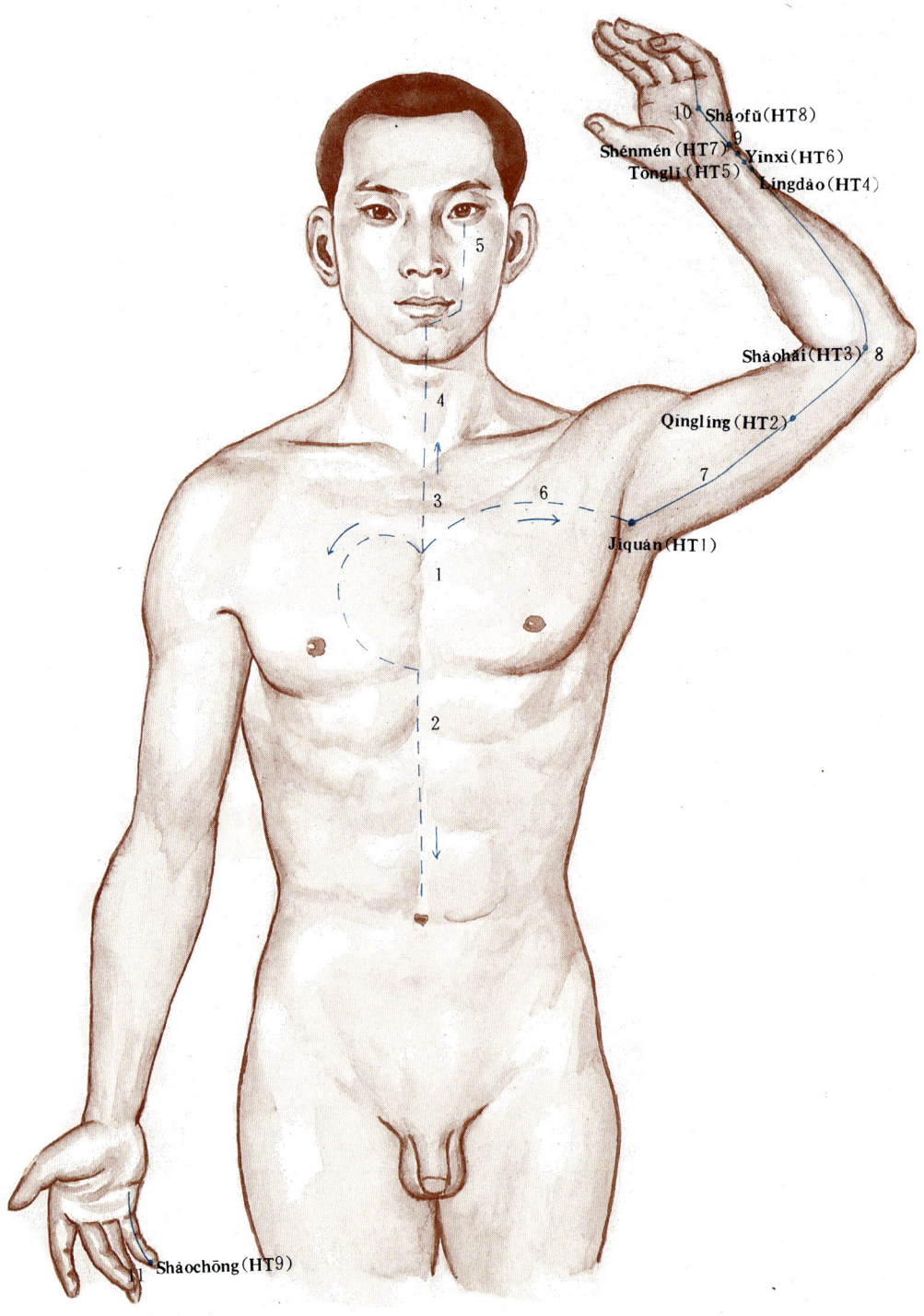

Fig. 7

(1) Course

This channel starts from the heart, comes out of the cardiac system (the large vessels connecting with other viscera) and descends through the diaphragm to connect with the small intestine.

The branch of the channel sprouts from the cardiac system, runs upwards along the side of the throat, and joins the ocular connectors (the structures connecting the eyeball with the brain, including blood vessels and optic nerves).

The original channel ascends to the axilla. And then it travels along the posterior border of the medial aspect of the upper arm, passes behind the Lung Channel of Hand-Taiyin and the Pericardium Channel of Hand-Jueyin, goes downwards and reaches the cubital fossa. It continues to run along the posterior border of the little finger reaches the tip (Point Shaochong, HT9), and finally connects with the Small Intestine Channel of Hand-Taiyang.

(2) Points of the Heart Meridian of Hand-Shaoyin, HT

Jiquan(HT1)

Location: At the apex of the axillary fossa, where the pulsation of the axillary artery is palpable.

Indications: Precordial pain, pain in the chest and hypochondriac region, scrofula, cold pain in the elbow and arm, dry throat.

Qingling(HT2)

Location: On the medial side of the arm and on the line connecting Jiquan(HT1) and Shaohai(HT3), 3 cun above the cubital crease, in the groove medial to the biceps muscle of the arm.

Indications: Precordial pain, pain in the shoulder, arm and hypochondriac region.

Shaohai(HT3)

Location: With the elbow flexed, at the midpoint of the line connecting the medial end of the cubital crease and the medial epicondyle of the humerus.

Indications: Precordial pain, contraction and numbness of the upper limb, tremor of the hand, scrofula, pain in the axillary and hypochondriac region.

Lingdao(HT4)

Location: On the palmar side of the forearm and on the radial side of the tendon of the ulnar flexor muscle of the wrist, 1.5 cun proximal to the crease of the wrist.

Indications: Precordial pain, contraction and pain of upper arm, sudden loss of voice, clonic convulsion.

Tongli(HT5)

Location: On the palmar side of the forearm and on the radial side of the tendon of the ulnar flexor muscle of the wrist, 1 cun proximal to the crease of the wrist.

Indications: Palpitation, dizziness, sore-throat, sudden loss of voice, stiffness of tongue, pain in the elbow and arm.

Yinxi(HT6)

Location: On the palmar side of the forearm and on the radial side of the tendon of the ulnar flexor muscle of the wrist, 1 cun proximal to the crease of the wrist.

Indications: Precordial pain, palpitation, hectic fever with night sweat, hematemesis, epistaxis, sudden loss of voice.

Shenmen(HT7)

Location: On the wrist, at ulnar end of the crease of the wrist, in the depression of the radial side of the tendon of the ulnar flexor muscle of the wrist.

Indications: Precordial pain, irritability, palpitation, amnesia, insomnia, manic-depressive psychosis, epilepsy, dementia, pain in the hypochondriac region, feverish sensation in palms, jaundice.

Shaofu(HT8)

Location: In the palm, between the 4th and 5th metacarpal bones, at the part of the palm touching the tip of the little finger when a fist is made.

Indications: Palpitation, chest pain, contraction of the little finger, feverish sensation in palms, enuresis, bradyuria, pruritus vulvae.

Shaochong(HT9)

Location: On the radial side of the distal segment of the little finger, 0.1 cun from the corner of the nail.

Indications: Palpitation, precordial pain, pain in the chest and hypochondriac region, manic-depressive psychosis, fever, coma.

6. The Small Intestine Meridian of Hand-Taiyang

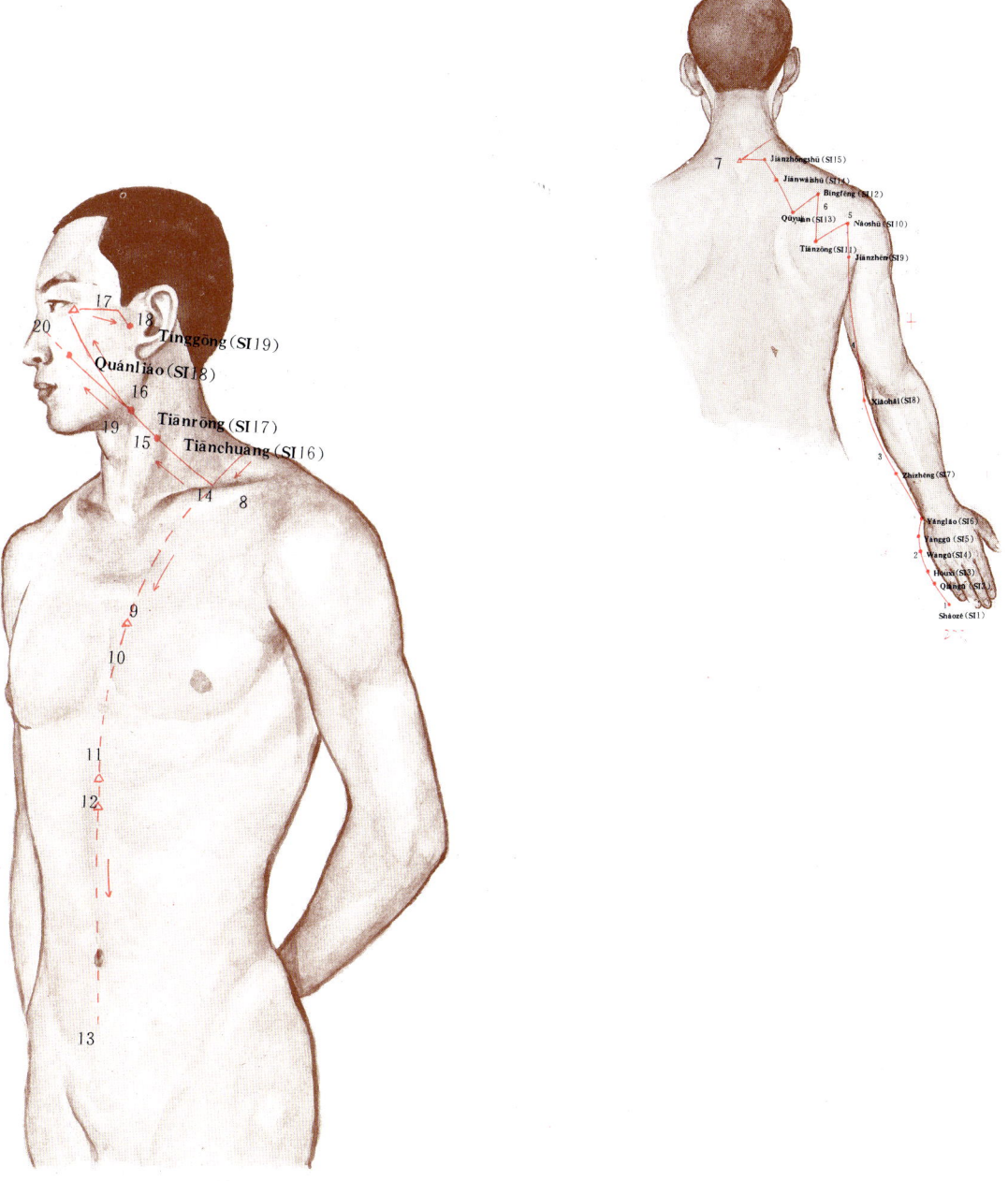

Fig. 8

(1) Course

This channel starts from the tip of the ulnar side of the little finger (Point Shaoze, SI1), and follows the ulnar border of the dorsum of the hand, ascends to the wrist, and then through the styloid process of the ulna and the posterior border of the forearm, finally passing between the olecranon of the ulna and the medial epicondyle of the humerus. It continues to travel along the posterior border of the lateral aspect of the upper arm, and out of the shoulder joint. Then circling round the shoulder-blade, it meets the Du Channel at Point Dazhui (DU14). From there it goes forward into the supraclavicular fossa and then connects with the heart. Descending along esophagus, it passes the diaphragm, reaches the stomach, and enters its pertaining organ, the small intestine.

One of the branches of this channel emerges from the supraclavicular fossa, and ascends along the neck to the cheek. From there it reaches the outer canthus of the eye, and then goes into the ear (at Point Tinggong, SI19).

The other branch of the channel, which is separated from the cheek, ascends to the infra-orbital region (Point Quanliao, SI18), reaches the lateral side of the nose and terminates at the inner canthus. Then it is distributed obliquely over the zygoma and connects with the Urinary Bladder Channel of Foot-Taiyang.

(2) Points of the Small Intestine Meridian of Hand-Taiyang, SI

Shaoze(SI1)

Location: On the ulnar side of the distal segment of the little finger, 0.1 cun from the corner of the nail.

Indications: Headache, fever, coma, lack of lactation, sore-throat, conjunctivitis.

Qiangu(SI2)

Location: At the junction of the red and white skin along the ulnar border of the hand, at the ulnar end of the crease of the 5th metacarpophslangeal joint when a loose fist is made.

Indications: Numbness of the fingers, fever, tinnitus, headache, dark urine.

Houxi(SI3)

Location: At the junction of the red and white skin along the ulnar border of the hand, at the ulnar end of the distal palmar crease, proximal to the 5th metacarpophalangeal joint when a hollow fist is made.

Indications: Stiffness of the nape, tinnitus and deafness, sore-throat, manic-depressive psychosis, malarial disease, sudden sprain in the lumbar region, fever with night sweat, numbness and contraction of the fingers, pain in the shoulder andarm.

Wangu(SI4)

Location: On the ulnar border of the hand, in the depression between the proximal end of the 5th metacarpal bone and hamate bone, and at the junction of the red and white skin.

Indications: Fever with anhidrosis, headache, stiffness of nape, contraction of fingers and carpal pain, jaundice.

Yanggu(SI5)

Location: On the ulnar border of the wrist, in the depression between the styloid process of thee ulna and triangular bone.

Indications: Swelling in the neck and submental region, carpal pain, fever.

Yanglao(SI6)

Location: On the ulnar side of the posterior surface of the forearm, in the depression proximal to and on the radial side of the head of the ulna.

Indications: Blurring of vision, pain in the elbow, shoulder and arm.

Zhizheng(SI7)

Location: On the ulnar side of the posterior surface of the forearm and on the line connecting Yanggu(SI5) and Xiaohai(SI8), 5 cun proximal to the dorsal crease of the wrist.

Indications: Stiffness of nape, headache, dizziness, contraction of elbow, arm and fingers, fever, manic-depressive psychosis.

Xiaohai(SI8)

Location: On the medial side of the elbow, in the depression between the olecranon of the ulna and the medial epicondyle of the humerus.

Indications: Headache, submental swelling, cervicodynia, pain in the shoulder, elbow and forearm, epilepsy.

Jianzhen(SI9)

Location: Posterior and inferior to the shoulder joint, 1 cun above the posterior end of the axillary fold with the arm adducted.

Indications: Pain in the scapular region, inability to raise arm.

Naoshu(SI10)

Location: On the shoulder, above the posterior end of the axillary fold, in the depression below the lower border of the scapular spine.

Indications: Swelling pain in the shoulder, aching pain and weakness in the shoulder and arm.

Tianzong(SI11)

Location: On the scapula, in the depression of the centre of the subscapular fossa, and on the level of the 4th thoracic vertebra.

Indication: Scapular pain, pain in the lateral part of the upper arm and elbow, dyspnea.

Bingfeng(SI12)

Location: On the scapula, at the centre of the suprascapular fossa, directly above Tianzong(SI11), in the depression found when the arm is raised.

Indications: Scapular pain, aching pain and numbness of the arm, inability to raise arm.

Quyuan(SI13)

Location: On the scapula, at the medial end of the suprascapular fossa, at the midpoint of the line connecting Naoshu(SI10) and the spinous process of the 2nd thoracic vertebra.

Indications: Contracting pain in the scapular region.

Jianwaishu(SI14)

Location: On the back, below the spinous process of the 1st thoracic vertebra, 3 cun lateral to the posterior midline.

Indications: Aching pain in the shoulder and back, stiffness of the neck and nape.

Jianzhongshu(SI15)

Location: On the back, below the spinous process of the 7th cervical vertebra, 2 cun lateral to the posterior midline.

Indications: cough with dyspnea, aching pain in the shoulder and back, hemoptysis.

Tianchuang(SI16)

Location: On the lateral side of the neck, posterior to the sternocleidomastoid muscle and Futu(LI18), on the level of the laryngeal protuberance.

Indications: Sore-throat, sudden loss of voice, deafness, tinnitus, stiffness of the neck and nape.

Tianrong(SI17)

Location: On the lateral side of the neck, posterior to the mandibular angle, in the depression of the anterior border of the sternocleidomastoid muscle.

Indications: Deafness, tinnitus, sore throat, swelling of the submental region, globus hystericus, goiter due to Qi disorders.

Quanliao(SI18)

Location: On the face, directly below the outer canthus, in the depression below the zygomatic bone.

Indications: Facial hemiparalysis, twitching of eyelid, prosopodynia, toothache, swelling of cheek, jaundice.

Tinggong(SI19)

Location: On the face, anterior to the tragus and posterior to the mandibular condyloid process, in the depression found when the mouth is open.

Indications: Deafness, tinnitus, otitis media suppurativa, dyscinesia of maxillary joint, toothache.

7. The Urinary Bladder Meridian of Foot-Taiyang

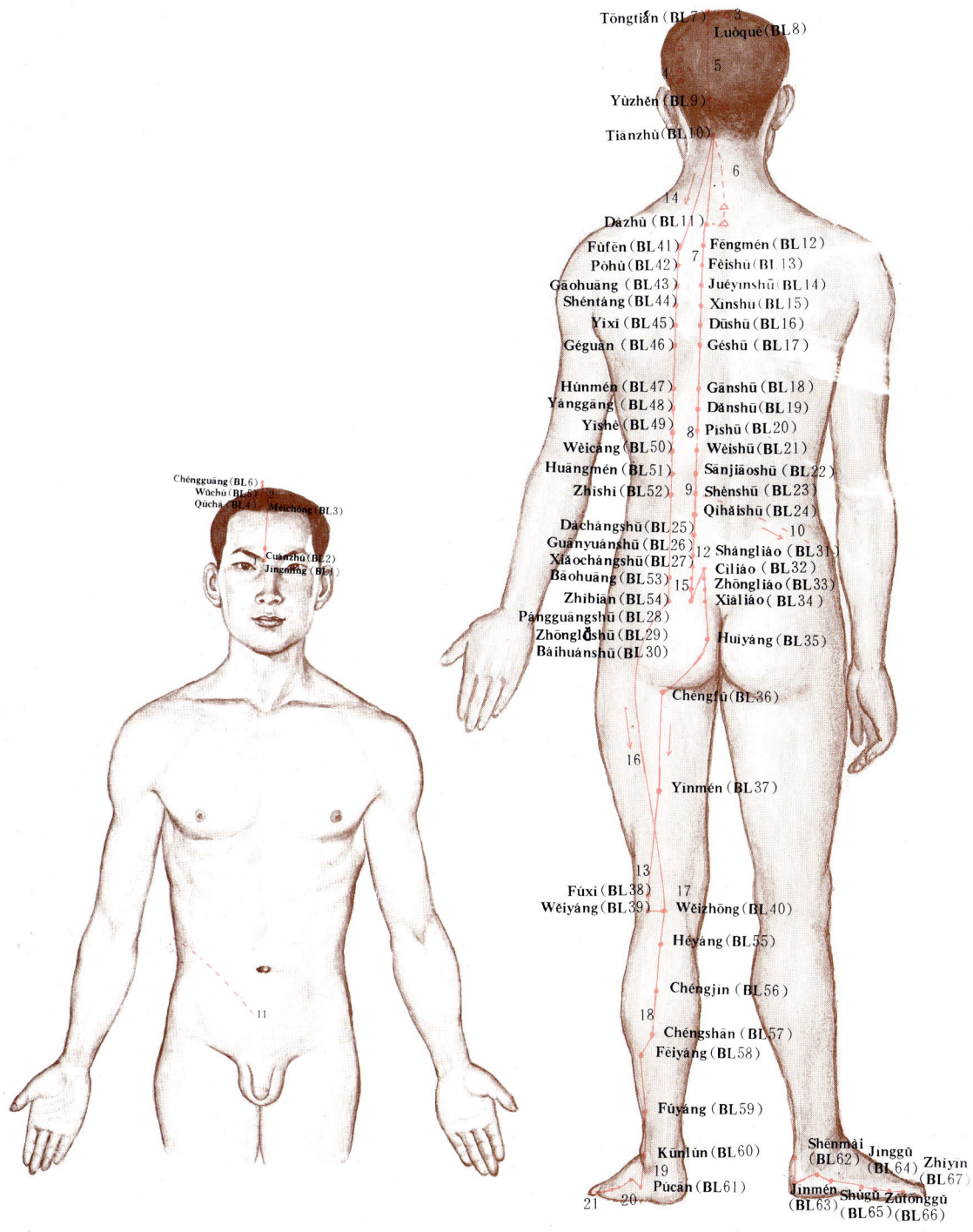

Fig. 9

(1) Course

This channel commences from the inner canthus, ascends to the forehead and joins its symmetrical channel at the vertex (Point Baihui, DU20).

One of its branches splits off the vertex and goes to the upper aspect of the auricle.

The original channel leaves the vertex for the brain where it re-emerges and runs downward to the back of the neck. Continuing along the medial side of the scapula, it travels parallel to the vertebral column and reaches the lumbar region. Passing the paravertebral muscles, it communicates with the kidney and enters into its pertaining organ, the urinary bladder.

The branch from the lumbar region runs downwards parallel to the vertebral column (1.5 individual cun lateral to the back mid-line), through the gluteal region, and into the popliteal fossa.

Another branch emerges from the original channel at the back of the neck, from the medial side of the scapula passes through the scapula, and runs down-parallel to the vertebral column (3 cun lateral to the back mid-line). Then it runs through the trochanter major of the femur, downwards along the posterior border of the lateral side of the thigh where it meets the branch descending from the lumbar region in the popliteal fossa. From there, it makes its way down through the musculus gastrocnemius, emerges from the posterior aspect of the external malleolus, runs along Point Jinggu(BL64) to the lateral side of the tip of the small toe (Point Zhiyin, BL67), where it connects with the Kidney Channel of Foot-Shaoyin.

(2) Points of the Bladder Meridian of Foot-Taiyang, BL

Jingming(BL1)

Location: On the face, in the depression slightly above the inner canthus.

Indications: Conjunctival congestion, ophthalmalgia, itching of the paropia, epiphora, night blindness, monochromatism, dizziness, myopia.

The patient is told to close his eyes when pushing gently the eyeball to the lateral side and fixing it with the left hand. Puncture slowly perpendicularly 0.1-1.0 cun with the right hand. It is not advisable to twirl or lift and thrust the needle. To avoid bleeding, press the puncturing site for 1-2 minutes after withdrawal of the needle, moxibustion is not used.

Cuanzhu(BL2)

Location: On the face, in the depression of the medial end of the eyebrow, at the supraorbital notch.

Indications: Headache, dizziness, orbital pain, blindness, epiphora, conjunctival congestion and ophthalmalgia, twitching of eyelid, optic atrophy.

Meichong(BL3)

Location: On the head, directly above Cuanzhu(BL2), 0.5 cun above the anterior hairline, on the line connecting Shenting(DU24) and Qucha(BL4)

Indications: Headache, dizziness, epilepsy, stuffy nose.

Qucha(BL4)

Location: On the head, 0.5 cun directly above the midpoint of the anterior hairline and 1.5 cun lateral to the midline, at the junction of the medial third and middle third of the line connecting Shenting(DU24) and Touwei(ST8).

Indications: Headache, stuffy nose, epistaxis, blurred vision, vertigo.

Wuchu(BL5)

Location: On the head, 1 cun directly above the midpoint of the anterior hairline and 1.5 cun lateral to the midline.

Indications: Headache, vertigo, epilepsy, clonic convulsion.

Chengguang(BL6)

Location: On the head, 2.5 cun directly above the midpoint of the anterior hairline and 1.5 cun lateral to the midline.

Indications: Headache, vertigo, stuffy nose.

Tongtian(BL7)

Location: On the head, 4 cun directly above the midpoint of the anterior hairline and 1.5 cun lateral to the midline.

Indications: Headache, dizziness, stuffy nose, epistaxis, rhinorrhea with turbid discharge.

Luoque(BL8)

Location: On the head, 5.5 cun directly above the midpoint of the anterior hairline and 1.5 cun lateral to the midline.

Indications: Vertigo, blurred vision, tinnitus, manic-depressive psychosis.

Yuzhen(BL9)

Location: On the occiput, 2.5 cun directly above the midpoint of the posterior hairline and 1.3 cun lateral to the midline, in the depression on the level of the upper border of the external occipital protuberance.

Indications: Headache radiating to the nape, dizziness, ophthalmalgia, stuffy nose.

Tianzhu(BL10)

Location: On the nape, in the depression of the lateral border of the trapezius muscle and 1.3 cun lateral to the midpoint of the posterior hairline.

Indications: Headache, stuffy nose, sore-throat, stiffness of nape, pain in the shoulder and back.

Dazhu(BL11)

Location: On the back, below the spinous process of the 1st thoracic vertebra, 1.5 cun lateral to the posterior midline.

Indications: Headache, pain in the nape and back, aching pain in the scapular region, cough, fever, stiffness of neck and nape.

Fengmen(BL12)

Location: On the back, below the spinous process of the 2nd thoracic vertebra, 1.5 cun lateral to the posterior midline.

Indications: Cough after catching cold, fever, headache, stiffness of nape, pain in the back and lumbar region.

Feishu(BL13)

Location: On the back, below the spinous process of the 3rd thoracic vertebra, 1.5 cun lateral to the posterior midline.

Indications: Cough with dyspnea, chest pain, hematemesis, hectic fever with night sweat.

Jueyinshu(BL14)

Location: On the back, below the spinous process of the 4th thoracic vertebra, 1.5 cun lateral to the posterior midline.

Indications: Cough, precordial pain, palpitation, chest distress, vomiting.

Xinshu(BL15)

Location: On the back, below the spinous process of the 5th thoracic vertebra, 1.5 cun lateral to the posterior midline.

Indications: Precordial pain, palpitation, amnesia, irritability, cough, hematemesis, emission, night sweat, manic-depressive psychosis, epilepsy.

Dushu(BL16)

Location: On the back, below the spinous process of the 6th thoracic vertebra, 1.5 cun lateral to the posterior midline.

Indications: Precordial pain, stomachache.

Geshu(BL17)

Location: On the back, below the spinous process of the 7th thoracic vertebra, 1.5 cun lateral to the posterior midline.

Indications: Vomiting, hiccup, dysphagia, cough with dyspnea, hematemesis, hectic fever with night sweat, rubella.

Ganshu(BL18)

Location: On the back, below the spinous process of the 8th thoracic vertebra, 1.5 cun lateral to the posterior midline.

Indications: Jaundice, pain in the hypochondriac region, vertigo, night blindness, manic-depressive psychosis, epilepsy, backache, hematemesis, epistaxis.

Danshu(BL19)

Location: On the back, below the spinous process of the 9th thoracic vertebra, 1.5 cun lateral to the osterior midline.

Indications: Jaundice, bitter taste, pain in the chest and hypochondriac region, consumption, hectic fever.

Pishu(BL20)

Location: On the back, below the spinous process of the 11th thoracic vertebra, 1.5 cun lateral to the posterior midline.

Indications: Epigastric pain, distention of the abdomen, jaundice, vomiting, diarrhea, dysentery, hematochezia, menorrhagia, edema, poor appetite, backache.

Weishu(BL21)

Location: On the back, below the spinous process of the 12th thoracic vertebra, 1.5 cun lateral to the posterior midline.

Indications: Pain in the chest and hypochondriac region, epigastric pain, anorexia, distention of the abdomen, borborygmus, diarrhea, nausea and vomiting.

Sanjiaoshu(BL22)

Location: On the low back, below the spinous process of the 1st lumbar vertebra, 1.5 cun lateral to the posterior midline.

Indications: Distention of the abdomen, borborygmus, indigestion, vomiting, diarrhea, dysentery, edema, stiffness and pain in the back.

Shenshu(BL23)

Location: On the low back, below the spinous process of the 2nd lumbar vertebra, 1.5 cun lateral to the posterior midline.

Indications: Emission, impotence, enuresis, irregular menstruation, leukorrhagia, lumbago, soreness and weakness of the waist and knee, dizziness and vertigo, tinnitus, deafness, edema, dyspnea, diarrhea.

Qihaishu(BL24)

Location: On the low back, below the spinous process of the 3rd lumbar vertebra, 1.5 cun lateral to the posterior midline.

Indications: Lumbago, irregular menstruation, dysmenorrhea, dyspnea.

Dachangshu(BL25)

Location: On the low back, below the spinous process of the 4th lumbar vertebra, 1.5 cun lateral to the posterior midline.

Indications: Aching pain in the back and lumbar region, distention of the abdomen, diarrhea, constipation, flaccidity of the lower extremities, lumbago and scelalgia.

Guanyuanshu(BL26)

Location: On the low back, below the spinous process of the 5th lumbar vertebra, 1.5 cun lateral to the posterior midline.

Indications: Lumbago, distention of abdomen, diarrhea, enuresis, scelalgia, frequency of micturition.

Xiaochangshu(BL27)

Location: On the sacrum and on the level of the 1st posterior sacral foramen, 1.5 cun lateral to the median sacral crest.

Indications: Distending pain in the lower abdomen, dysentery, emission, hematuresis, enuresis, leukorrhagia, lumbosacral pain, lumbago and scelalgia.

Pangguangshu(BL28)

Location: On the sacrum and on the level of the 2nd posterior sacral foramen, 1.5 cun lateral to the median sacral crest.

Indications: Interrupted urination, enuresis, frequency of micturition, diarrhea, constipation, stiffness and pain in the back and lumbar region.

Zhonglushu(Bl29)

Location: On the sacrum and on the level of the 3rd posterior sacral foramen, 1.5 cun lateral to the median sacral crest.

Indications: Dysentery, hernia, stiffness of the back.

Baihuanshu(BL30)

Location: On the sacrum and on the level of the 4th posterior sacral foramen, 1.5 cun lateral to the median sacral crest.

Indications: Enuresis, severe abdominal pain accompanied by difficulty of urination and constipation, abnormal vaginal discharge, irregular menstruation, cold pain in lumbo-iliac region, dysuria and dysphoria, rectal tenesmus, proctoptosis

Shangliao(BL31)

Location: On the sacrum, at the midpoint between the posterosuperior iliac spine and the posterior midline, just at the 1st posterior sacral foramen.

Indications: Lumbago, dysuria and dysphoria, irregular menstruation, abnormal vaginal discharge, prolapse of uterus.

Ciliao(BL32)

Location: On the sacrum, medial and inferior to the posterosuperior iliac spine, just at the 2nd posterior sacral foramen.

Indications: Lumbago, hernia, irregular menstruation, abnormal discharge, dysmenorrhea, emission, impotence, enuresis, dysuria, flaccidity of lower extremities.

Zhongliao(BL33)

Location: On the sacrum, medial and inferior to the posterosuperior iliac spine, just at the 3rd posterior sacral foramen.

Indications: Lumbago, constipation, diarrhea, enuresis, irregular menstruation, leukorrhagia.

Xialiao(BL34)

Location: On the sacrum, medial and inferior to the posterosuperior iliac spine, just at the 4th posterior sacral foramen.

Indications: Lumbago, pain in the lower abdomen, dysuria, constipation, leukorrhagia.

Huiyang(BL35)

Location: On the sacrum, 0.5 cun lateral to the tip of the coccyx.

Indications: Dysentery, hematochezia, diarrhea, hemorrhoid, impotence, leukorrhagia.

Chengfu(BL36)

Location: On the posterior side of the thigh, at the midpoint of the inferior gluteal crease.

Indications: Lumbosacral pain radiating to the buttock and thigh, flaccidity of the lower extremities, dysphoria, hemorrhoid.

Yinmen(BL37)

Location: On the posterior side of the thigh on the line connecting Chengfu(BL36) and Weizhong(BL40), 6 cun below Chengfu(BL36).

Indications: Lumbago and scelalgia, flaccidity or paralysis of the lower extremities.

Fuxi(BL38)

Location: At the lateral end of the popliteal crease, 1 cun above Weiyang(BL39), medial to the tendon of the biceps muscle of the thigh.

Indications: Numbness of the buttock and thigh, systremma.

Weiyang(BL39)

Location: At the lateral end of the popliteal crease, medial to the tendon of the biceps muscle of the thigh.

Indications: Stiffness of the back and lumbar region, distention of the lower abdomen, edema, dysuria, contraction of the leg and foot.

Weizhong(BL40)

Location: At the midpoint of the popliteal crease, between the tendon of the biceps muscle of the thigh and the semitendinous muscle.

Indications: Lumbago, dyscinesia of the hip joint, systremma, flaccidity of lower extremities, hemiparalysis, vomiting and diarrhea, erysipelas.

Fufen(BL41)

Location: On the back, below the spinous process of the 2nd thoracic vertebra, 3 cun lateral to the posterior midline.

Indications: Contraction of the shoulder and back, stiffness of the neck and nape, numbness of the elbow and forearm.

Pohu(BL42)

Location: On the back, below the spinous process of the 3rd thoracic vertebra, 3 cun lateral to the posterior midline.

Indications: Consumption, cough with dyspnea, hemoptysis, stiffness of the nape, pain in the shoulder and back.

Gaohuang(BL43)

Location: On the back, below the spinous process of the 4th thoracic vertebra, 3 cun lateral to the posterior midline.

Indications: Consumption, cough with dyspnea, hemoptysis, night sweat, amnesia, emission.

Shentang(BL44)
Location: On the back, below the spinous process of the 5th thoracic vertebra, 3 cun lateral to the posterior midline.

Indications: Dyspnea, precordial pain, palpitation, chest distress, cough, stiffness of the back.

Yixi(BL45)
Location: On the back, below the spinous process of the 6th thoracic vertebra, 3 cun lateral to the posterior midline.

Indications: Cough, dyspnea, pain in the shoulder and back.

Geguan(BL46)
Location: On the back, below the spinous process of the 7th thoracic vertebra, 3 cun lateral to the posterior midline.

Indications: Difficulty in eating and drinking because of ascending of stomach-Qi, hiccup, vomiting, eructation, stiffness of the back.

Hunmen(BL47)
Location: On the back, below the spinous process of the 9th thoracic vertebra, 3 cun lateral to the posterior midline.

Indications: Pain in the chest and hypochondriac region, backache, vomiting, diarrhea.

Yanggang(BL48)
Location: On the back, below the spinous process of the 10th thoracic vertebra, 3 cun lateral to the posterior midline.

Indications: Borborygmus, abdominal pain, diarrhea, pain in the hypochondriac region, jaundice.

Yishe(BL49)
Location: On the back, below the spinous process of the 11th thoracic vertebra, 3 cun lateral to the posterior midline.

Indications: Distention of the abdomen, borborygmus, vomiting, diarrhea, difficulty in eating and drinking because of ascending of stomach-Qi.

Weicang(BL50)
Location: On the back, below the spinous process of the 12th thoracic vertebra, 3 cun lateral to the posterior midline.

Indications: Distention of the abdomen, epigastric pain, backache, infantile indigestion with food retention.

Huangmen(BL51)
Location: On the low back, below the spinous process of the 1st lumbar vertebra, 3 cun lateral to the posterior midline.

Indications: Abdominal pain, constipation, mass in the abdomen.

Zhishi(BL52)
Location: On the low back, below the spinous process of the 2nd lumbar vertebra, 3 cun lateral to the posterior midline.

Indications: Emission, impotence, enuresis, frequency of micturition, irregular menstruation, aching pain in the waist and knee, edema.

Baohuang(BL53)
Location: On the buttock and on the level of the 2nd posterior sacral foramen, 3 cun lateral to the median sacral crest.

Indications: Borborygmus, distention of the abdomen, backache and lumbago, anuresis.

Zhibian(BL54)

Location: On the buttock and on the level of the 4th posterior sacral foramen, 3 cun lateral to the median sacral crest.

Indications: Lumbosacral pain, flaccidity of the lower extremities, dysuria, swelling pain in the vulvae, hemorrhoid, dyschezia.

Heyang(BL55)

Location: On the posterior side of the leg and on the line connecting Weizhong (BL40) and Chengshan(BL57), 2 cun below Weizhong(BL40).

Indications: Lumbago and backache, Aching pain and numbness of the lower extremities.

Chengjin(BL56)

Location: On the posterior side of the leg and on the line connecting Weizhong(BL40) and Chengshan(BL57), at the centre of the gastrocnemius muscle belly, 5 cun below Weizhong(BL40).

Indications: Scelalgia and myospasm, hemorrhoid, contraction of the back and waist.

Chengshan(BL57)

Location: On the posterior midline of the leg, between Weizhong(BL40) and Kunlun(BL60), in a pointed depression formed below the gastrocnemius muscle belly when the leg is stretched or the heel is lifted.

Indications: Lumbago, scelalgia, systremma, myospasm, hemorrhoid, constipation, beriberi.

Feiyang(BL58)

Location: On the posterior side of the leg, 7 cun directly above Kunlun(BL60) and 1 cun lateral and inferior to Chengshan(BL57).

Indications: Headache, vertigo, stuffy nose, nasal bleeding, lumbago, hemorrhoid, weakness of the lower extremities.

Fuyang(BL59)

Location: On the posterior side of the leg, posterior to the lateral malleolus, 3 cun directly above Kunlun(BL60).

Indications: Lightheadedness, headache, lumbosacral pain, swelling pain in the lateral malleolus, paralysis of the lower extremities.

Kunlun(BL60)

Location: Posterior to the lateral malleolus, in the depression between the tip of the external malleolus and Achilles tendon.

Indications: Headache, vertigo, stiffness of the nape, epistaxis, pain in the shoulder, lumbago and scelalgia, painful heels, dystocia, epilepsy.

Pucan(BL61)

Location: On the lateral side of the foot, posterior and inferior to the external malleolus, directly below Kunlun (BL60), lateral to the calcaneum, at the junction of the red and white skin.

Indications: Flaccidity of the lower extremities, painful heels.

Shenmai(BL62)

Location: On the lateral side of the foot, in the depression directly below the external malleolus.

Indications: Epilepsy, manic-depressive psychosis, headache, dizziness, insomnia, aching pain in the lumbocrural region.

Jinmen(BL63)

Location: On the lateral side of the foot, directly below the anterior border of the external malleolus, on the lower border of the cuboid bone.

Indications: Manic-depressive psychosis, epilepsy, infantile convulsion, lumbago, pain in the lateral malleolus, numbness and pain in the lower extremities.

Jinggu(BL64)

Location: On the lateral side of the foot, below the tuberosity of the 5th metatarsal bone, at the junction of the red and white skin.

Indications: Headache, stiffness of the nape, lumbocrural pain, epilepsy.

Shugu(BL65)

Location: On the lateral side of the foot, posterior to the 5th metatarsophalangeal joint, at the junction of the red and white skin.

Indications: Manic-depressive psychosis, headache, stiffness of the nape, vertigo, lumbago, pain in the posterior portion of the lower extremities.

Zutonggu(BL66)

Location: On the lateral side of the foot, anterior to the 5th metatarsophalangeal joint, at the junction of the red and white skin.

Indications: Headache, stiffness of the nape, vertigo, epistaxis, manic-depressive psychosis.

Zhiyin(BL67)

Location: On the lateral side of the distal segment of the little toe, 0.1 cun from the corner of the toenail.

Indications: Headache, stuffy nose, nasal bleeding, ophthalmalgia, malposition of fetus, dystocia, retention of placenta.

8. The Kidney Meridian of Foot-Shaoyin

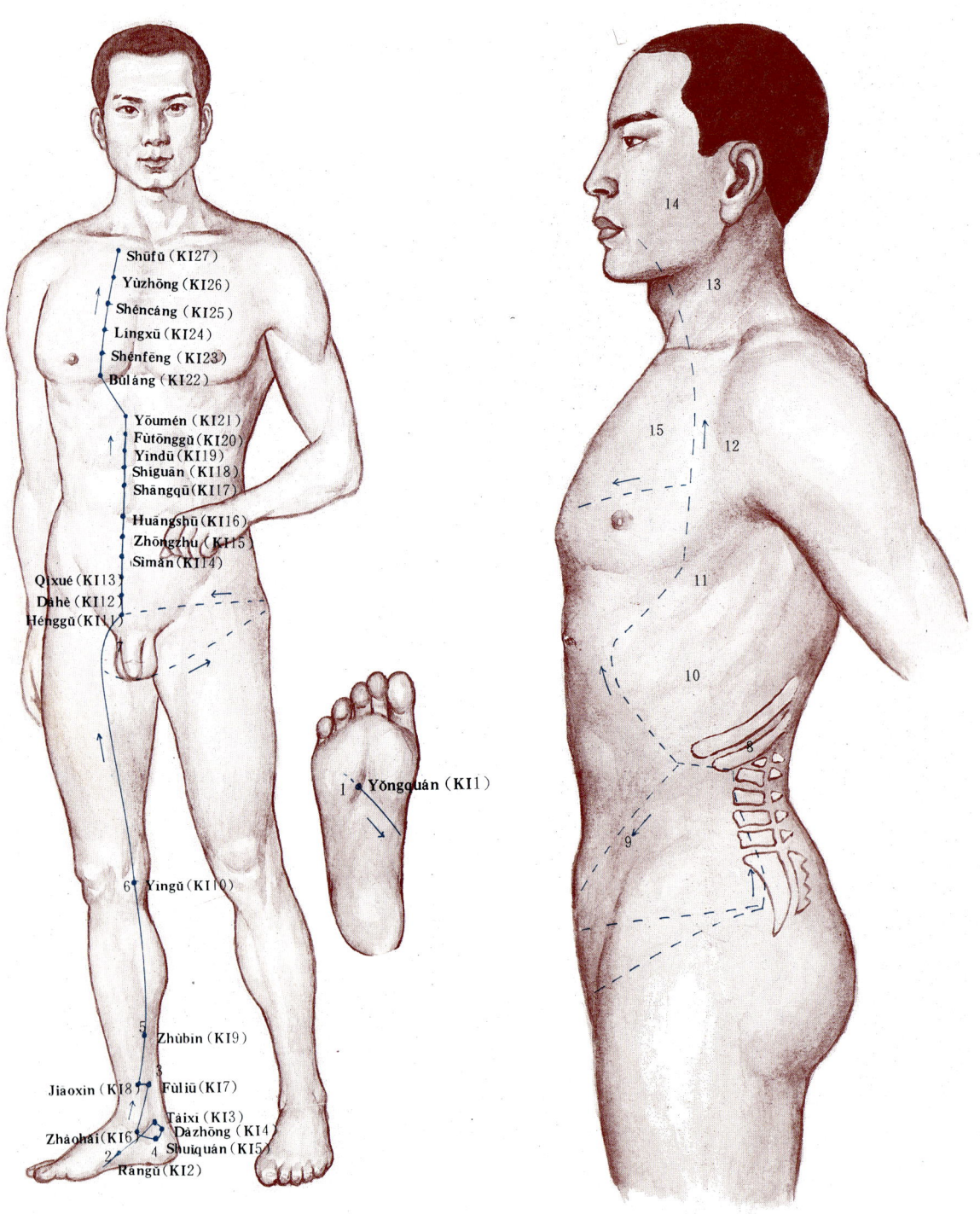

Fig. 10

(1) Course

The Kidney Channel of Foot-Shaoyin starts from the plantar surface of the little toe, and runs obliquely towards the center of he sole of the foot (Point Yongquan, KI1). Emerging from Point Rangu (KI2), the interior aspect of the tuberosity of the navicular bone, it runs behind the medial malleolus, and reaches the heel. Then it ascends along the medial side of the popliteal fossa. Ascending continuously along the medio-posterior aspect of the thigh, it runs through the vertebral column. From there it enters its pertaining organ, the kidney, and communicates with the urinary bladder.

Its direct branch re-emerges from the kidney, runs straight up through the kidney, runs straight up through the liver and diaphragm, into the lung, from which it travels along the throat and terminates at the root of the tongue.

Another branch of its exits from the lung, connects with the heart, and is distributed over the thoracic cavity to meet with the Pericardium Channel of Hand-Jueyin.

(2) Points of the Kidney Meridian Of Foot-Shaoyin, KI

Yongquan(KI1)

Location: On the sole, in the depression appearing on the anterior part of the sole when the foot is in the plantar flexion, approximately at the junction of the anterior third and posterior two-thirds of the line connecting the base of the 2nd and 3rd toes and the heel.

Indications: Headache, vertigo, dizziness, sore-throat, dry tongue, aphonia, dyschezia, dysuria, infantile convulsion, feverish sensation in the soles, coma.

Rangu(KI2)

Location: On the medial border of the foot, below the tuberosity of the navicular bone, and at the junction of the red and white skin.

Indications: Pruritus vulvae, prolapse of uterus, irregular menstruation, emission, hemoptysis, diabetes, diarrhea, swelling pain in the dorsum pedis, tetanus neonatorum.

Taixi(KI3)

Location: On the medial border of the foot, posterior to the medial malleolus, in the depression between the tip of the medial malleolus and Achilles tendon.

Indications: Dry and sore throat, toothache, deafness, tinnitus, dizziness, hemoptysis, dyspnea, diabetes, irregular menstruation, insomnia, emission, impotence, frequency of micturition, lumbago.

Dazhong(KI4)

Location: On the medial border of the foot, posterior and inferior to the medial malleolus, in the depression of the medial side of and anterior to the attachment of the Achilles tendon.

Indications: Hemoptysis, dyspnea, stiffness of the back and lumbar region, dysuria and dyschezia, painful heels, dementia.

Shuiquan(KI5)

Location: On the medial border of the foot, posterior and inferior to the medial malleolus, 1 cun directly below Taixi(KI3). In the depression of the medial side of the tuberosity of the calcaneum.

Indications: Amenorrhea, irregular menstruation, dysmenorrhea, prolapse of uterus, dysuria, blurred vision.

Zhaohai(KI6)

Location: On the medial border of the foot, in the depression below the tip of the medial malleolus.

Indications: Irregular menstruation, abnormal vaginal discharge, prolapse of uterus, pruritus vulave, frequency of micturition, anuresis, constipation, epilepsy, insomnia, dry and sore throat, dyspnea.

Fuliu(KI7)

Location: On the medial side of the leg, 2 cun directly above Taixi(KI3) , anterior to the Achilles tendon.

Indications: edema, distention of the abdomen, borborygmus, weakness of the lower extremities, night sweat, spontaneous perspiration, fever with anhidrosis.

Jiaoxin(KI8)

Location: On the medial side of the leg, 2 cun above Taixi(KI3) and 0. 5 cun anterior to Fuliu(KI7), posterior to the medial border of the tibia.

Indications: Irregular menstruation, dysmenorrhea, metrorrhagia and metrostaxis, prolapse of uterus, diarrhea, constipation, swelling pain in the testes.

Zhubin(KI9)

Location: On the medial side of the leg and on the line connecting Taixi(KI3) and Yingu(KI10), 5 cun above Taixi(KI3) , medial and inferior to the gastrocnemius muscle belly.

Indications: Manic-depressive psychosis, pain in the foot and leg, pain due to hernia.

Yingu(KI10)

Location: On the medial side of the popliteal fossa, between the tendons of the semitendinous and semimembranous muscles when the knee is flexed.

Indications: Impotence, pain due to hernia, metrorrhagia and metrostaxis, dysuria, aching pain in the knee, manic-depressive psychosis.

Henggu(KI11)

Location: On the lower abdomen, 5 cun below the centre of the umbilicus and 0. 5 cun lateral to the anterior midline.

Indications: Distending pain in the lower abdomen, dysuria, enuresis, emission, impotence, vulval pain.

Dahe(KI12)

Location: On the lower abdomen, 4 cun below the centre of the umbilicus and 0. 5 cun lateral to the anterior midline.

Indications: Emission, impotence, leukorrhagia, vulval pain, prolapse of uterus.

Qixue(KI13)

Location: On the lower abdomen, 3 cun below the centre of the umbilicus and 0. 5 cun lateral to the anterior midline.

Indications: Irregular menstruation, dysmenorrhea, dysuria, abdominal pain, diarrhea.

Siman(KI14)

Location: On the lower abdomen, 2 cun below the centre of the umbilicus and 0. 5 cun lateral to the anterior midline.

Indications: Distention of the abdomen, pain in the abdomen, diarrhea, emission, emission, irregular menstruation, dysmenorrhea, postpartum abdominal pain.

Zhongzhu(KI15)

Location: On the lower abdomen, 1 cun below the centre of the umbilicus and 0. 5 cun lateral to the anterior midline.

Indications: Irregular menstruation, abdominal pain, constipation.

Huangshu(KI16)

Location: On the middle abdomen, 0.5 cun lateral to the centre of the umbilicus.

Indications: Abdominal pain, distention in the abdomen, vomiting, constipation, diarrhea.

Shangqu(KI17)

Location: On the upper abdomen, 2 cun above the centre of the umbilicus, and 0.5 cun lateral to the anterior midline.

Indications: Abdominal pain, diarrhea, constipation.

Shiguan(KI18)

Location: On the upper abdomen, 3 cun above the centre of the umbilicus, and 0.5 cun lateral to the anterior midline.

Indications: Vomiting, abdominal pain, constipation, postpartum abdominal pain, sterility.

Yindu(KI19)

Location: On the upper abdomen, 4 cun above the centre of the umbilicus, and 0.5 cun lateral to the anterior midline.

Indications: Borborygmus, abdominal pain, epigastric pain, constipation, vomiting.

Futonggu(KI20)

Location: On the upper abdomen, 5 cun above the centre of the umbilicus, and 0.5 cun lateral to the anterior midline.

Indications: Abdominal pain, distention of the abdomen, vomiting, indigestion.

Youmen(KI21)

Location: On the upper abdomen, 6 cun above the centre of the umbilicus, and 0.5 cun lateral to the anterior midline.

Indications: Abdominal pain, distention of the abdomen, indigestion, vomiting, diarrhea, morning sick or hyperemesis gravidarum.

Bulang(KI22)

Location: On the chest, in the 5th intercostal space, 2 cun lateral to the anterior midline.

Indications: Cough with dyspnea, distention of the chest and hypochondriac region, vomiting, anorexia.

Shenfeng(KI23)

Location: On the chest, in the 4th intercostal space, 2 cun lateral to the anterior midline.

Indications: Cough with dyspnea, distention of the chest and hypochondriac region, mastitis.

Lingxu(KI24)

Location: On the chest, in the 3th intercostal space, 2 cun lateral to the anterior midline.

Indications: Cough with dyspnea, distention of the chest and hypochondriac region, mastitis.

Shencang(KI25)

Location: On the chest, in the 2th intercostal space, 2 cun lateral to the anterior midline.

Indications: Cough with dyspnea, chest pain.

Yuzhong(KI26)

Location: On the chest, in the 1st intercostal space, 2 cun lateral to the anterior midline.

Indications: Cough with dyspnea, accumulation of phlegm, distention of the chest and hypochondriac region.

Shufu(KI27)

Location: On the chest, below the lower border of the clavicle, 2 cun lateral to the anterior midline.

Indications: Cough with dyspnea, chest pain.

9. The Pericardium Meridian of Hand-Jueyin

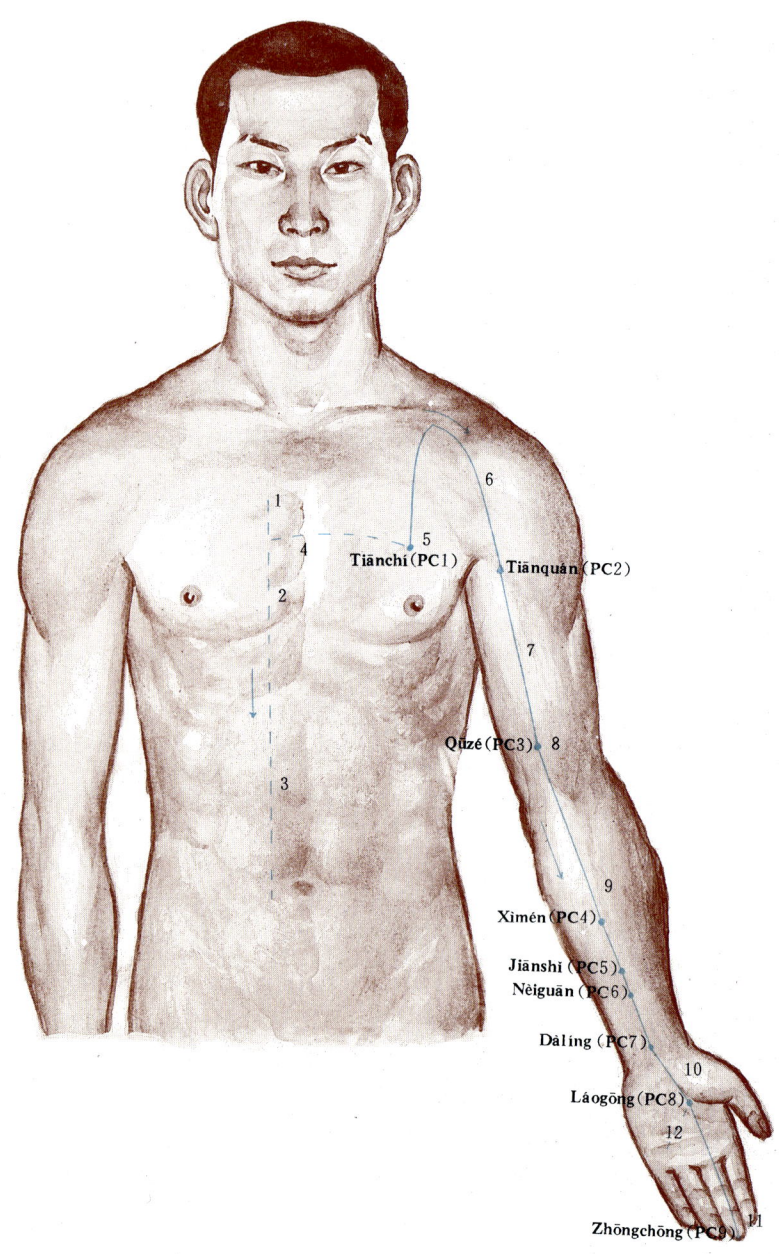

Fig. 11

(1) Course

This channel commences from the chest where it exits from its pertaining organ, the pericardium. Then it descends through the diaphragm and links up with the triple warmers in the upper, the middle and the lower portions of the body cavity.

One of its branches runs along the chest, through the costal region at a point 3 cun below the armpit, and ascends to the axilla. From the medial aspect of the upper arm, it makes its way downwards between the Lung Channel and the Heart Channel, and reaches the cubital fossa. From there it runs still further downwards to the forearm between the tendons of m. palmaris longus and m. flexorcarpi, and enters the palm. It runs along the middle finger to its tip (Point Zhongchong, PC9).

Another branch of its leaves the palm (Point Laogong, PC8), runs along the ring finger to its tip (Point Guanchong, SJ1), and connects with the Triple Warmer Channel of Hand-Shaoyang.

(2) Points of the Pericardium Meridian of Hand-Jueyin, PC

Tianchi(PC1)

Location: On the chest, in the 4th intercostal space, 1 cun lateral to the nipple and 5 cun lateral to the anterior midline.

Indications: Chest distress, pain in the hypochondriac region, swelling pain in the axillary fossa.

Tianquan(PC2)

Location: On the medial side of the arm, 2 cun below the anterior end of the axillary fold, between the long and short heads of the biceps muscle of the arm.

Indications: Precordial pain, distention of the hypochondriac region, cough, pain in the thoracic wall and medial portion of the upper arm.

Quze(PC3)

Location: At the midpoint of the cubital crease, on the ulnar side of the tendon of the biceps muscle of the arm.

Indications: Precordial pain, palpitation, fever, irritability, stomachache, vomiting, aching pain in the elbow and forearm, tremor of the forearm and hand.

Ximen(PC4)

Location: On the palmar side of the forearm and on the line connecting Quze(PC3) and Daling(PC7), 5 cun above the crease of the wrist.

Indications: Precordial pain, palpitation, epistaxis, hematemesis, hemoptysis, chest pain, furuncle, epilepsy.

Jianshi(PC5)

Location: On the palmar side of the forearm and on the line connecting Quze(PC3) and Daling(PC7), 3 cun above the crease of the wrist.

Indications: Precordial pain, palpitation, stomachache, vomiting, fever, irritability, malaria, manic-depressive psychosis, epilepsy, swelling of axillary region, contraction of the elbow and arm.

Neiguan(PC6)

Location: On the palmar side of the forearm and on the line connecting Quze(PC3) and Daling(PC7), 2 cun above the crease of the wrist.

Indications: Precordial pain, palpitation, chest distress, pain in the hypochondriac region, vomiting and nausea, hiccup, manic-depressive psychosis, epilepsy, insomnia, fever, irritability, malaria, contraction of the elbow and arm.

Daling(PC7)

Location: At the midpoint of the crease of the wrist, between the tendons of the long palmar muscle and radial flexor muscle of the wrist.

Indications: Precordial pain, palpitation, stomachache, vomiting, manic-depressive psychosis, epilepsy, chest distress, pain in the hypochondriac region, palpitation, insomnia, irritability, ozostomia.

Laogong(PC8)

Location: At the centre of the palm, between the 2nd and 3rd metacarpal bones, but close to the latter, and in the part touching the tip of the middle finger when a fist is made.

Indications: Precordial pain, manic-depressive psychosis, epilepsy, aphthae, ozostomia, tinea unguium, vomiting and nausea.

Zhongchong(PC9)

Location: At the centre of the tip of the middle finger.

Indications: Precordial pain, irritability, coma, swelling pain and stiffness of the tongue, fever, heat stroke, convulsion, feverish sensation in the palms.

10. The Triple Warmer Sanjiao Meridian of Hand-Shaoyang

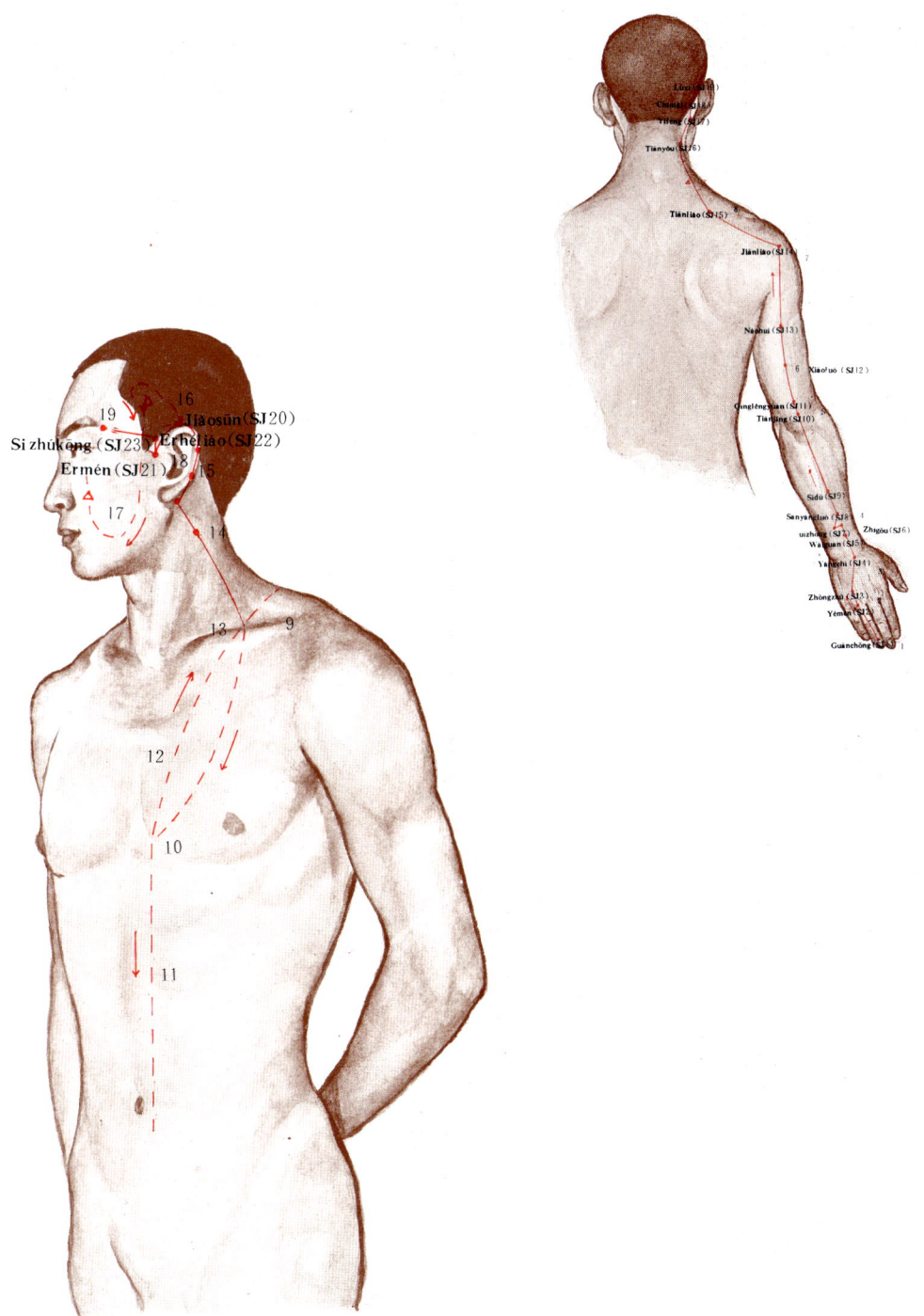

Fig. 12

(1) Course

The Triple Warmer Channel of Hand-Shaoyang starts from the ulnar side of the tip of the ring finger (Point Guanchong, SJ1), and runs upwards between the two fingers i. e., the 4th and 5th metacarpal bones. Along the dorsum of the wrist, it travels to the dorsal side of the forearm between the two bones or the radius and ulna. It goes upwards through the olecranon, along the lateral aspect of the upper arm, to the shoulder region, where it meets the Gall Bladder Channel of Foot-Shaoyang, and afterwards leaves its posterior aspect for the supraclavicular fossa. From the fossa it descends arther, is distributed to Point Danzhong (RN17), or the region in the centre between the two breasts, and communicates with the pericardium. Descending through the diaphragm, it reaches the triple warmer, i. e. the upper, middle and lower portions of the body cavity in succession.

One of its branches originates from Point Shanzhong (RN17) and ascends to the supraclavicular fossa, from where it goes upwards to the nape of the neck. From the posterior border of the ear, it makes a direct ascent through the superior aspect of the auricula, curves down the cheek, and then reaches the infraorbital region.

Another branch originates in the retro-auricular region and passes into the ear. Emerging in front of the ear, it runs in front of Point Shangguan(GB3), across the above-mentioned branch at the cheek and reaches the outer canthus, where it connects with the Gall Bladder Channel of Foot-Shaoyang.

(2) Points of the Sanjiao Meridian of Hand-Shaoyang, SJ

Guanchong(SJ1)

Location: On the ulnar side of the distal segment of the 4th finger, 0. 1 cun from the corner of the nail.

Indications: Headache, conjunctival congestion, sore-throat, stiffness of the tongue, fever, irritability.

Yemen(SJ2)

Location: On the dorsum of the hand, between the 4th and 5th fingers, at the junction of the red and white skin, proximal to the margin of the web.

Indications: Headache, conjunctival congestion, sore-throat, sudden deafness, malaria, brachialgia.

Zhongzhu(SJ3)

Location: On the dorsum of the hand, proximal to the 4th metacarpophalangeal joint, in the depression between the 4th and 5th metacarpal bones.

Indications: Headache, conjunctival congestion, sore-throat, deafness, tinnitus, fever, brachialgia, stiffness of the fingers.

Yangchi(SJ4)

Location: At the midpoint of the dorsal crease of the wrist, in the depression on the ulnar side of the tendon of the extensor muscle of the fingers.

Indications: Pain in the shoulder and arm, pain in the wrist, malaria, deafness, diabetes.

Waiguan(SJ5)

Location: On the dorsal side of the forearm and on the line connecting Yangchi (SJ4) and the tip of the olecranon, 2 cun proximal to the dorsal crease of the wrist, between the radius and ulna.

Indications: Fever, headache, pain in the cheek, stiffneck, deafness, tinnitus, pain in the hypochondriac region, dyscinesia of the elbow, pain in the fingers, tremor of the hand.

Zhigou(SJ6)

Location: On the dorsal side of the forearm and on the line connecting Yangchi(SJ4) and the tip of the olecranon, 3 cun proximal to the dorsal crease of the wrist, between the radius and ulna.

Indications: Deafness, tinnitus, pain in the hypochondriac region, vomiting, constipation, fever, soreness and heaviness sensation in the shoulder and back, sudden loss of voice.

Huizong(SJ7)

Location: On the dorsal side of the forearm, 3 cun proximal to the dorsal crease of the wrist, on the ulnar side of Zhigou(SJ6) and on the radial border of the ulna.

Indications: Deafness, otalgia, epilepsy, brachialgia.

Sanyangluo(SJ8)

Location: On the dorsal side of the forearm, 4 cun proximal to the dorsal crease of the wrist, between the radius and the ulna.

Indications: Deafness, sudden loss of voice, pain in the chest and hypochondriac region, brachialgia, toothache.

Sidu(SJ9)

Location: On the dorsal side of the forearm and on the line connecting Yangchi(SJ4) and the tip of the olecranon, 5 cun distal to the tip of the olecranon, 5 cun distal to the tip of the olecranon, between the radius and ulna.

Indications: Deafness, toothache, migraine, sudden loss of voice, pain in the forearm.

Tianjing(SJ10)

Location: On the lateral side of the upper arm, in the depression 1 cun proximal to the tip of the olecranon when the elbow is flexed.

Indications: Migraine, pain in the neck, nape, shoulders and arms, epilepsy, scrofula, goiter due to Qi disorders.

Qinglengyuan(SJ11)

Location: With the elbow flexed, on the lateral side of the upper arm, 2 cun above the tip of the olecranon and 1 cun above Tianjing(SJ10).

Indications: Inability to raise arm due to pain in the shoulder and arm, migraine.

Xiaoluo(SJ12)

Location: On the lateral side of the upper arm, at the midpoint of the line connecting Qinglengyuan(SJ11) and Naohui(SJ13).

Indications: Headache, stiffness of the neck and nape, inability to raise arm due to brachialgia.

Naohui(SJ13)

Location: On the lateral side of the upper arm and on the line connecting the tip of the olecranon and Jianliao(SJ14), 3 cun below Jianliao(SJ14), and on the posteroinferior border of the deltoid muscle.

Indications: Goiter due to Qi disorders, aching pain in the shoulder and arm.

Jianliao(SJ14)

Location: On the shoulder, posterior to Jianyu(LI15), in the depression inferior and posterior to the acromion when the arm is abducted.

Indications: Inability to raise arm due to pain in the shoulder and arm, flaccidity of the upper limb.

Tianliao(SJ15)

Location: On the scapula, at the midpoint between Jianjing(GB21) and Quyuan(SI13), at the superior angle of the scapula.

Indications: Pain in the shoulder and elbow, stiffness of the neck and nape.

Tianyou(SJ16)

Location: On the lateral side of the neck, directly below the posterior border of the mastoid process, on the level of the mandibular angle, and on theposterior border of the sternocleidomastoid muscle.

Indications: Headache, stiffness of the nape, edema of face, blurred vision, sudden deafness.

Yifeng(SJ17)

Location: Posterior to the ear lobe, in the depression between the mastoid process and mandibular angle.

Indications: Tinnitus, deafness, otitis media suppurativa, facial hemiparalysis, toothache, swelling of the cheek, scrofula, dyscinesia of maxillary joint.

Chimai(SJ18)

Location: On the head, at the centre of the mastoid process, and at the junction of the middle third and lower third of the line connecting Jiaosun(SJ20) and Yifeng(SJ17) along the curve of the ear helix.

Indications: Headache, tinnitus, deafness, infantile convulsion and epilepsy.

Luxi(SJ19)

Location: On the head, at the junction of the upper third and middle third of the line connecting Jiaosun(SJ20) and Yifeng(SJ17) along the curve of the ear helix.

Indications: Headache, tinnitus, otalgia, deafness, infantile convulsion and epilepsy.

Jiaosun(SJ20)

Location: On the head, above the ear apex within the hairline.

Indications: Tinnitus, conjunctivitis, gingival swelling pain, toothache, mumps.

Ermen(SJ21)

Location: On the face, anterior to the supratragic notch, in the depression behind the posterior border of the condyloid process of the mandible.

Indications: Tinnitus, deafness, otitis media suppurativa, toothache.

Erheliao(SJ22)

Location: On the lateral side of the head, on the posterior margin of the temples, anterior to the anterior border of the root of the ear auricle and posterior to the superficial temporal artery.

Indications: Migraine, tinnitus, lockjaw.

Sizhukong(SJ23)

Location: On the face, in the depression of the lateral end of the eyebrow.

Indications: Headache, conjunctivitis, vertigo, twitching of eyelid, toothache, facial hemiparalysis.

11. The Gall Bladder Meridian of Foot-Shaoyang

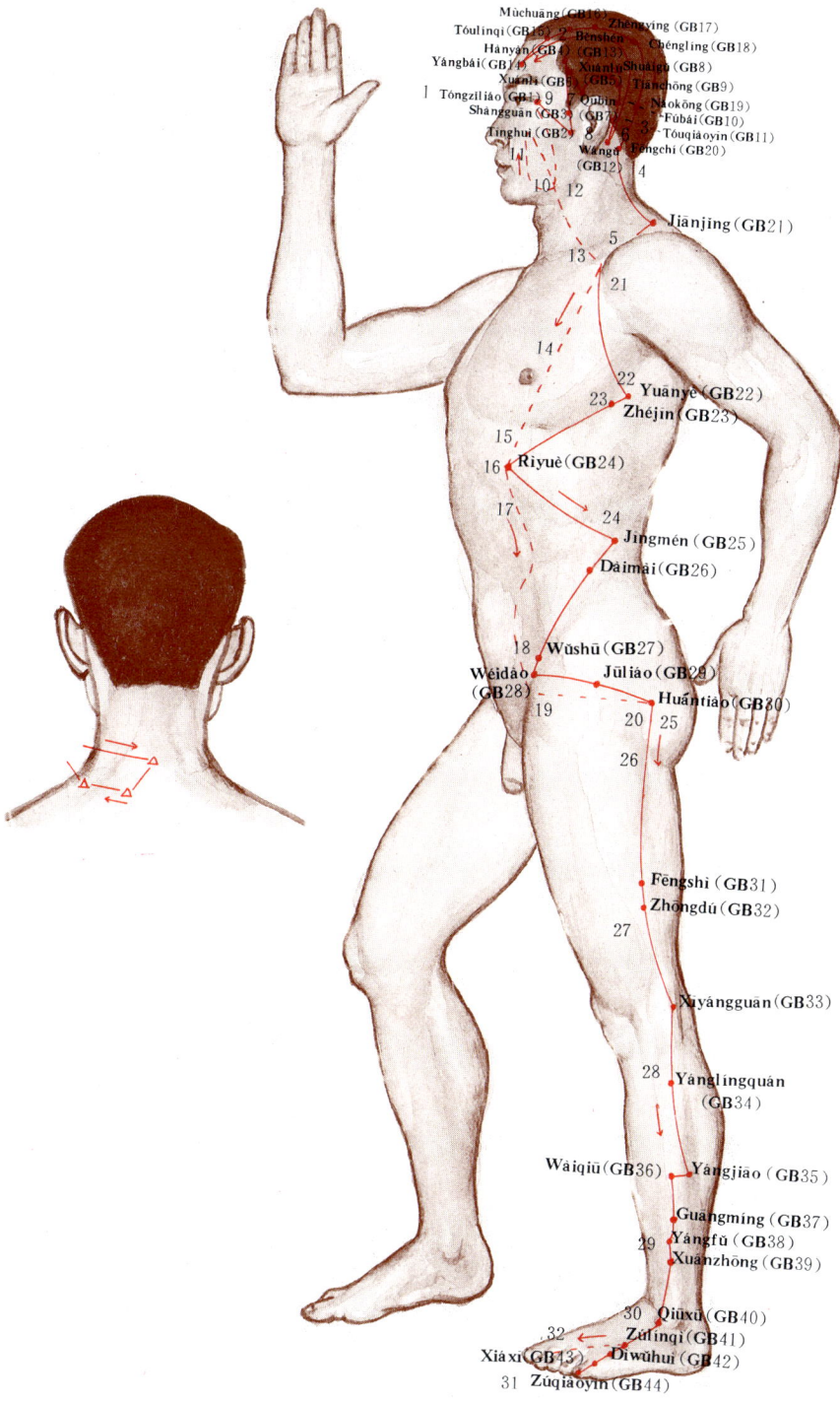

Fig. 13

(1) Course

This channel starts from the outer canthus of the eye, runs upwards to the corner of the forehead, and curves downwards to the retro-auricular region. Then it runs along the side of the neck in front of the Triple Warmer Channel to the shoulder. Turning backwards it goes behind the Triple Warmer Channel of Hand-Shaoyang, and enters the supraclavicular fossa.

One of its branches originates in the retro-auricular region, passes through the ear, re-emerges in front of the ear and then reaches the posterior aspect of the outer canthus of the eye.

Another branch leaves the outer canthus for Point Daying (ST5) and meets the Triple Warmer Meridian of Hand-Shaoyang again. From there it reaches the infraorbital region, then descends through Point Jiache(ST6) to the neck, from where it passes into the supraclavicular fossa and meets the original channel. The it continues to travel through the chest, the diaphragm, the liver, and then to the gall bladder. It then travels along the inside of the hypochondrium, through Point Qichong(ST30), around the margin of the pubisure, transversely into Point Huantiao (GB30).

A third straight branch descends from the supraclavicular fossa to the axilla, from where it continues its descent along the lateral aspect of the chest, through the hypochondrium, to Huantiao(GB30), and meets the above-mentioned branch. From Huantiao(GB30), it goes down along the lateral aspect of the thigh, emerges from the lateral side of the knee, and continues its downward travel along the anterior aspect of the fibula, and straight to Juegu, a hollow in the low part of the fibula and 3 individual cun above the external malleolus. Running further downwards, it emerges in front of the external malleolus. Along the dorsum of the foot, it finds its terminus at the lateral side of the tip of the 4th toe.

A fourth branch leaves the dorsum of the foot, makes its way first between the 1st and 2nd metatarsal bones, then through the distal portion of the big toe, back to its nail and finally out of the hair portion proximal to it, and communicates with the Liver Channel of Foot-Jueyin.

(2) Points of the Gallbladder Meridian of Foot-Shaoyang, GB

Tongziliao(GB1)

Location: On the face, lateral to the outer canthus, on the lateral border of the orbit.

Indications: Headache, conjunctivitis, epiphora, hypopsia, facial hemiparalysis.

Tinghui(GB2)

Location: On the face, anterior to the intertragic notch, in the depression posterior to the condyloid process of the mandible when the mouth is open.

Indications: Deafness, tinnitus, toothache, dyscinesia of maxillary joint, mumps, facial hemiparalysis.

Shangguan(GB3)

Location: Anterior to the ear, directly above Xiaguan(ST7), in the depression above the upper border of the zygomatic arch.

Indications: Headache, tinnitus, deafness, otitis media suppurativa, facial hemiparalysis, toothache.

Hanyan(GB4)

Location: On the head, in the hair above the temples, at the junction of the upper fourth and lower three fourths of the curved line connecting Touwei(ST8) and Qubin(GB7).

Indications: Migraine, vertigo, tinnitus, pain in the outer canthus, toothache, convulsion, epilepsy.

Xuanlu(GB5)

Location: On the head, in the hair above the temples, at the midpoint of the curved line connecting Touwei (ST8) and Qubin(GB7).

Indications: Migraine, pain in the outer canthus, edema of face.

Xuanli(GB6)

Location: On the head, in the hair above the temples, at the junction of the upper three fourths and lower fourth of the curved line connecting Touwei(ST8)and Qubin(GB7).

Indications: Migraine, pain in the outer canthus, tinnitus.

Qubin(GB7)

Location: On the head, at a crossing point of the vertical posterior border of the temples and horizontal line through the ear apex.

Indications: Migraine, swelling in the cheek and submental region, lockjaw, infantile convulsion.

Shuaigu(GB8)

Location: On the head, directly above the ear apex, 1.5 cun above the hairline, directly above Jiaosun(SJ20).

Indications: Migraine, dizziness, vomiting, infantile convulsion.

Tianchong(GB9)

Location: On the head, directly above the posterior border of the ear root, 2 cun above the hairline and 0.5 cun posterior to Shuaigu(GB8).

Indications: Headache, epilepsy, gingival swelling pain, fright.

Fubai(GB10)

Location: On the head, posterior and superior to the mastoid process, at the junction of the middle third and upper third of the curved line connecting Tianchong(GB9) and Wangu(GB12).

Indications: Headache, tinnitus, deafness.

Touqiaoyin(GB11)

Location: On the head, posterior and superior to the mastoid process, at the junction of the middle third and lower third of the curved line connecting Tianchong(GB9) and Wangu(GB12).

Indications: Headache radiating to the nape, otalgia, tinnitus, deafness.

Wangu(GB12)

Location: On the head, in the depression posterior and inferior to the mastoid process.

Indications: Headache, insomnia, swelling cheek, pain in the opisthotic region, facial hemiparalysis, toothache.

Benshen(GB13)

Location: On the head, 0.5 cun above the anterior hairline, 3 cun lateral to Shenting(DU24), at the junction of the medial two thirds and lateral third of the line connecting Shenting(DU24) and Touwei(ST8).

Indications: Headache, insomnia, vertigo, epilepsy.

Yangbai(GB14)

Location: On the forehead, directly above the pupil, 1 cun above the eyebrow.

Indications: pain in the forehead, orbital pain, ophthalmalgia, vertigo, twitching of the eyelid, blepharoptosis, epiphora.

Toulinqi(GB15)

Location: On the head, directly above the pupil and 0.5 cun above the anterior hairline, at the midpoint of the line connecting Shenting(DU24) and Touwei(ST8).

Indications: Headache, vertigo, epiphora, pain in the outer canthus, stuffy nose, rhinorrhea with turbid discharge.

Muchuang(GB16)
Location: On the head, 1.5 cun above the anterior hairline and 2.25 cun lateral to the midline of the head.

Indications: Headache, dizziness, conjunctivitis, stuffy nose.

Zhengying(GB17)
Location: On the head, 2.5 cun above the anterior hairline and 2.25 cun lateral to the midline of the head.

Indications: Migraine, dizziness.

Chengling(GB18)
Location: On the head, 4 cun above the anterior hairline and 2.25 cun lateral to the midline of the head.

Indications: Headache, dizziness, epistaxis, rhinorrhea with turbid discharge.

Naokong(GB19)
Location: On the head and on the level of the upper border of the external occipital protuberance or Naohu(DU17), 2.25 cun lateral to the midline of the head.

Indications: Headache, stiffness of nape, dizziness, ophthalmalgia, tinnitus, epilepsy.

Fengchi(GB20)
Location: On the nape, below the occipital bone, on the level of Fengfu(DU16), in the depression between the upper ends of the sternocleidomastoid and trapezius muscles.

Indications: Headache, dizziness, insomnia, stiffness of the neck and nape, blurring of vision, optic atrophy, conjunctivitis, tinnitus, convulsion, infantile convulsion, epilepsy, fever, common cold, stuffy nose, rhinorrhea with turbid discharge.

Jianjing(GB21)
Location: On the shoulder, directly above the nipple, at the midpoint of the line connecting Dazhui(DU14) and the acromion.

Indications: Stiffness of neck and nape, pain in the shoulder and arm, inability to raise, galactostasis, acute mastitis, scrofula, apoplexy, dystocia.

Yuanye(GB22)
Location: On the lateral side of the chest, on the midaxillary line when the arm is raised, 3 cun below the axilla, in the 4th intercostal space.

Indications: Chest distress, swelling of the axillary fossa, pain in the hypochondriac region, inability to raise arm due to brachialgia.

Zhejin(GB23)
Location: On the lateral side of the chest, 1 cun anterior to Yuanye(GB22), on the level of the nipple, and in the 4th intercostal space.

Indications: Chest distress, pain in the hypochondriac region, dyspnea.

Riyue(GB24)
Location: On the upper abdomen, directly below the nipple, in the 7th intercostal space, 4 cun lateral to the anterior midline.

Indications: Pain in the hypochondriac region, vomiting, acid regurgitation, hiccup, jaundice, mastitis.

Jingmen(GB25)
Location: On the lateral side of the waist, 1.8 cun posterior to Zhangmen(LR13), below the free end of the 12th rib.

Indications: Distention of the abdomen, borborygmus, diarrhea, lumbago and hypochondriac pain.

Daimai(GB26)

Location: On the lateral side of the abdomen, 1.8 cun below Zhangmen(LR13), at the crossing point of a vertical line through the free end of the 11th rib and a horizontal line through the umbilicus.

Indications: Irregular menstruation, amenorrhea, abnormal vaginal discharge, abdominal pain, hernia, lumbago and hypochondriac pain.

Wushu(GB27)

Location: On the lateral side of the abdomen, anterior to the anterosuperior iliac spine, 3 cun below the level of the umbilicus.

Indications: Abnormal vaginal discharge, lumbago and scelalgia, pain in the lower abdomen, hernia, constipation.

Weidao(GB28)

Location: On the lateral side of the abdomen, anterior and inferior to the anterosuperior iliac spine, 0.5 cun anterior and inferior to Wushu(GB27).

Indications: Leukorrhagia, pain in the lower abdomen, hernia, prolapse of uterus.

Juliao(GB29)

Location: On the hip, at the midpoint of the line connecting the anterosuperior iliac spine and the prominence of the great trochanter.

Indications: lumbago with numbness, paralysis, flaccidity of the lower extremities.

Huantiao(GB30)

Location: On the lateral side of the thigh, at the junction of the middle third and lateral third of the line connecting the prominence of the great trochanter and the sacral hiatus when the patient is in a lateral recumbent position with the thigh flexed.

Indications: Lumbago, numbness of the lower extremities, hemiparalysis.

Fengshi(GB31)

Location: On the lateral midline of the thigh, 7 cun above the popliteal crease, or at the place touching the tip of the middle finger when the patient stands erect with the arms hanging down freely.

Indications: Aching pain in the lumbocrural region, flaccidity of the lower extremities, prurigo universalis.

Zhongdu(GB32)

Location: On the lateral side of the thigh, 2 cun below Fengshi(GB31), or 5 cun above the popliteal crease, between the lateral vastus muscle and biceps muscle of the thigh.

Indications: Aching pain in the waist and knee, flaccidity and numbness of the lower extremities, hemiparalysis.

Xiyangguan(GB33)

Location: On the lateral side of the knee, 3 cun above Yanglingquan(GB34), in the depression above the external epicondyle of the femur.

Indications: Swelling pain in the knee, systremma, numbness of the leg.

Yanglingquan(GB34)

Location: On the lateral side of the leg, in the depression anterior and inferior to the head of the fibula.

Indications: Hemiparalysis, flaccidity and numbness of the lower extremities, swelling pain in the knee, beriberi, hypochondriac pain, bitter taste, vomiting, jaundice, infantile convulsion.

Yangjiao(GB35)

Location: On the lateral side of the leg, 7 cun above the tip of the external malleolus, on the posterior border of the fibula.

Indications: Distention of the chest and hypochondriac region, flaccidity of the lower extremities.

Waiqiu(GB36)

Location: On the lateral side of the leg, 7 cun above the tip of the external malleolus, on the anterior border of the fibula and on the level of Yangjiao(GB35).

Indications: Pain in the chest and hypochondriac region, pain in the neck and nape, pain in the lower extremities, rabies.

Guangming(GB37)

Location: On the lateral side of the leg, 5 cun above the tip of the external malleolus, on the anterior border of the fibula.

Indications: Gonalgia, flaccidity of the lower extremities, blurred vision, ophthalmalgia, night blindness, distending pain in the breast.

Yangfu(GB38)

Location: On the lateral side of the leg, 4 cun above the tip of the external malleolus, on the anterior border of the fibula.

Indications: Migraine, pain in the outer canthus, swelling in the axillary fossa, scrofula, lumbago, pain in the chest and hypochondriac region, pain in the lateral portion of the lower extremities, malaria.

Xuanzhong(GB39)

Location: On the lateral side of the leg, 3 cun above the tip of the external malleolus, on the anterior border of the fibula.

Indications: Hemiparalysis due to apoplexy, pain in the neck and nape, distention of the abdomen, hypochondriac pain, flaccidity of the lower extremities, myospasm of the leg and foot, beriberi.

Qiuxu(GB40)

Location: Anterior and inferior to the external malleolus, in the depression lateral to the tendon of the long extensor muscle of the toes.

Indications: Pain in the neck and nape, swelling in the axillary region, pain in the chest and hypochondriac region, vomiting, regurgitation of acid, flaccidity of the lower extremities, swelling pain in the lateral malleolus, malaria.

Zulinqi(GB41)

Location: On the lateral side of the instep of the foot, posterior to the 4th metatarsophalangeal joint, in the depression lateral to the tendon of the extensor muscle of the little toe.

Indications: Headache, dizziness, pain in the outer canthus, scrofula, pain in the chest and hypochondriac region, distending pain in the breast, irregular menstruation, swelling pain in the dorsum of the foot, contracting pain in the toe(s).

Diwuhui(GB42)

Location: On the lateral side of the instep of the foot, posterior to the 4th metatarsophalangeal joint, between the 4th and 5th metatarsal bones, medial to the tendon of the extensor muscle of the little toe.

Indications: Pain in the canthus, tinnitus, distending pain in the breast, swelling pain in the dorsum of the foot.

Xiaxi(GB43)

Location: On the lateral side of the Instep of the foot, between the 4th and 5th toes, at the junction of the red and white skin, proximal to the margin of the web.

Indications: Headache, dizziness, pain in the outer canthus, tinnitus, deafness, edema of the cheek, pain in the chest and hypochondriac region, fever.

Zuqiaoyin(GB44)

Location: On the lateral side of the distal segment of the 4th toe, 0.1 cun from the corner of the toenail.

Indications: Headache, tinnitus, deafness, ophthalmalgia, dreaminess, fever.

12. The Liver Meridian of Foot-Jueyin

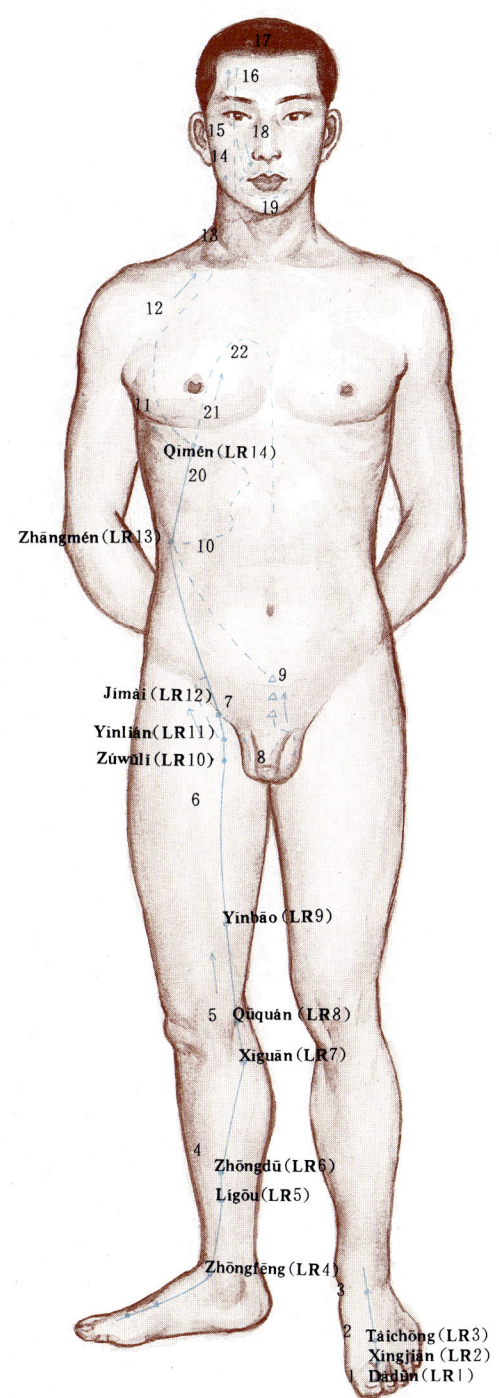

Fig. 14

(1) Course

The Liver Channel of Foot-Jueyin starts from the border of the hair behind the nail of the great toe, passes the dorsum of the foot and reaches the region one individual cun in front of the medial malleolus. From there, it ascends 8 individual cun above the medial malleolus where it crosses the Spleen Meridian of Foot-Taiyin, then runs behind the channel up to the medial border of the popliteal fossa. It continues its ascent along the medial side of the thigh, to the pubic region where it curves round the external genitalia and enters the lower abdomen. From there, it runs upwards via the stomach into its pertaining organ, the liver, and communicates with the gall bladder. Further upward, it passes through the diaphragm, is distributed to the hypochondrium, and ascends along the posterior aspect of the larynx to the nasopharynx, where it connects with the surrounding tissues of the eye, then emerges from the forehead, and finally meets the Du Channel at the vertex.

One of its branches originates in the tissues connecting the eye ball with the brain, goes downwards into the cheek and curves round the inner surface of the lips.

Another branch originates in the liver, passes through the diaphragm and penetrates to the lung, where it connects with the Lung Channel of Hand-Taiyin.

(2) Points of the Liver Meridian of Foot-Jueyin, LR

Dadun(LR1)

Location: On the lateral side of the distal segment of the great toe, 0.1 cun from the corner of the toenail.

Indications: Hernia, enuresis, metrorrhagia and metrostaxis, prolapse of the uterus, epilepsy.

Xingjian(LR2)

Location: On the instep of the foot, between the 1st and 2nd toes, at the junction of the red and white skin proximal to the margin of the web.

Indications: Headache, dizziness, night blindness, thirst, hypochondriac pain, distention of the abdomen, pain due to hernia, dysuria, urodynia, irregular menstruation, epilepsy, insomnia, convulsion.

Taichong(LR3)

Location: On the instep of the foot, in the depression of the posterior end of the 1st interosseous metatarsal space.

Indications: Headache, dizziness, insomnia, conjunctival congestion accompanied with swelling pain, melancholia, infantile convulsion, thirst, hypochondriac pain, metrorrhagia and metrostaxis, hernia, enuresis, dysuria, epilepsy, pain in the anterior margin of the medial malleolus.

Zhongfeng(LR4)

Location: On the instep of the foot, anterior to the medial malleolus, on the line connecting Shangqiu(SP5) and Jiexi(ST41), in the depression medial to the tendon of the anterior tibial muscle.

Indications: Pain due to hernia, pudendal pain, emission, dysuria, distending pain in the chest and hypochondriac region.

Ligou(LR5)

Location: On the medial side of the leg, 5 cun above the tip of the medial malleolus, on the midline of the medial surface of the tibia.

Indications: Dysuria, enuresis, hernia, irregular menstruation, morbid leukorrhes, pruritus vulvae, flaccidity of the lower limbs.

Zhongdu(LR6)

Location: On the medial side of the leg, 7 cun above the tip of the medial malleolus, on the midline of the medial surface of the tibia.

Indications: Pain in the abdomen and hypochondriac region, diarrhea, hernia, metrorrhagia and metrostaxis, lochiorrhea.

Xiguan(LR7)

Location: On the medial side of the leg, posterior and inferior to the medial epicondyle of the tibia, 1 cun posterior to Yinlingquan(SP9), at the upper end of the medial head of the gastrocnemius muscle.

Indications: Gonalgia.

Ququan(LR8)

Location: On the medial side of the knee, at the medial end of the popliteal crease when the knee is flexed, posterior to the medial epicondyle of the tibia, in the depression of the anterior border of the insertions of the semimembranous and semitnedinous muscles.

Indications: Pain in the lower abdomen, dysuria, emission, pain in the vulvae, prolapse of uterus, pruritus vulvae, pain in the medial portion of the thighand knee.

Yinbao(LR9)

Location: On the medial side of the thigh, 4 cun above the medial epicondyle of the femur, between the medial vastus muscle and sartorius muscle.

Indications: Lumbosacral pain radiating to the lower abdomen, dysuria, enuresis, irregular menstruation.

Zuwuli(LR10)

Location: On the medial side of the thigh, 3 cun directly below Qichong(ST30), at the proximal end of the thigh below the pubic tubercle and on the lateral border of the long abductor muscle of the thigh.

Indications: Distention of the lower abdomen, retention of urine.

Yinlian(LR11)

Location: On the medial side of the thigh, 2 cun directly below Qichong(ST30), at the proximal end of the thigh below the pubic tubercle and on the lateral border of the long abductor muscle of the thigh.

Indications: Irregular menstruation, morbid leukorrhage, pain in the lower abdomen, pain in the thigh.

Jimai(LR12)

Location: Lateral to the pubic tubercle, lateral and inferior to Qichong(ST30), in the inguinal groove where the pulsation of the femoral artery is palpable, 2.5 cun lateral to the anterior midline.

Indications: Pain in the lower abdominal region, pain in the vulva, hernia.

Zhangmen(LR13)

Location: On the lateral side of the abdomen, belwo the free end of the 11thrib.

Indications: Hypochondriac pain, distention of the abdomen, borborygmus, vomiting, diarrhea, indigestion.

Qimen(LR14)

Location: On the chest, directly below the nipple, in the 6th intercostal space, 4 cun lateral to the anterior midline.

Indications: Hypochondriac pain, distention of the abdomen, hiccup, regurgitation of acid, mastitis, melancholia.

13. The Du Channel

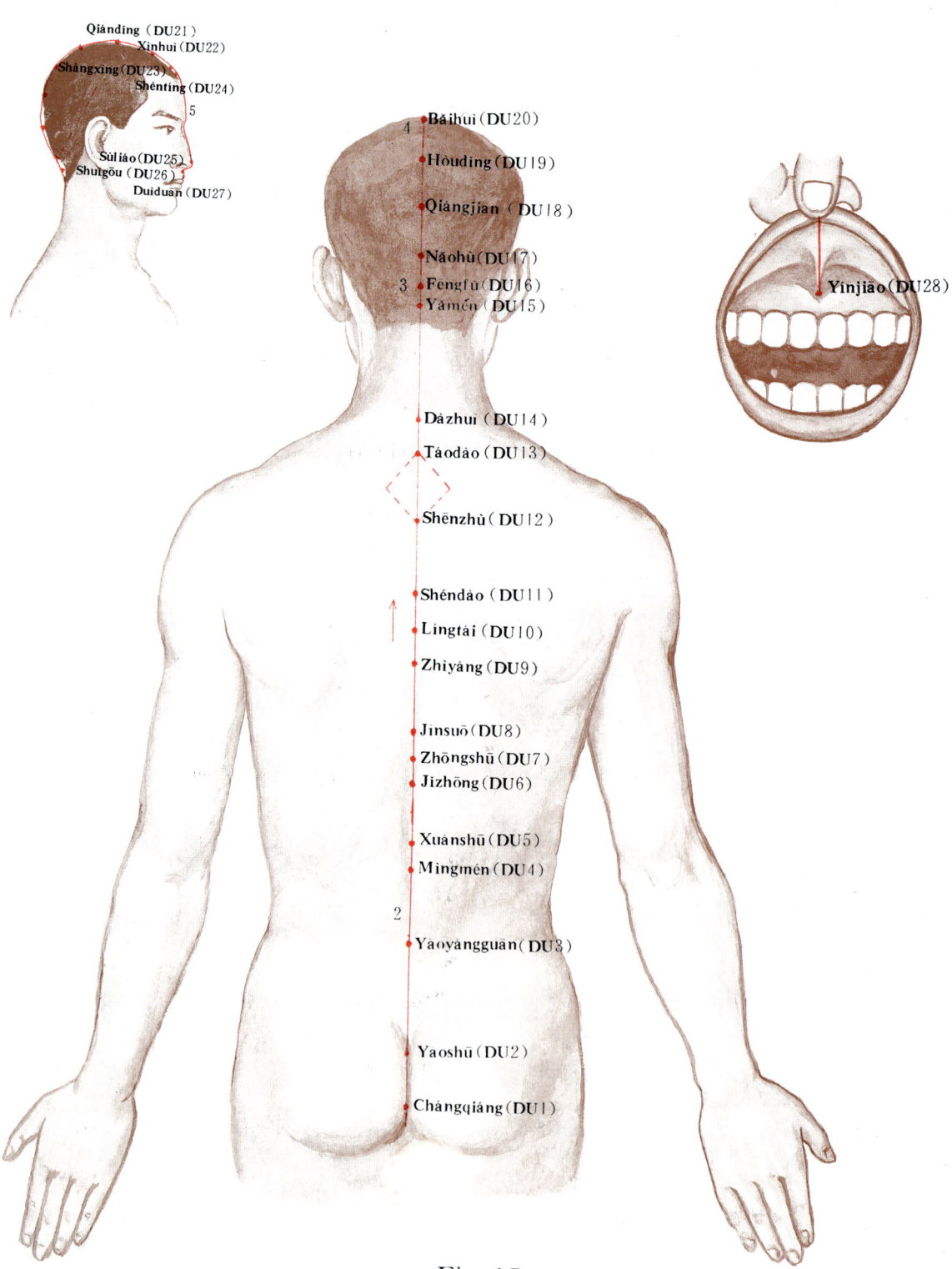

Fig. 15

The word "Du" in Chinese means " a general superintendent". The Du Channel runs along the midline of the back, and meets with the three Yang Channels of Hand and Foot as well as the Yangwei Channel several times in its course, and is able to superintend all yang channels of the body, so this channel is also named "the sea of the yang channels".

(1) Course

The channel originates in the lower part of the abdomen below the umbilicus, makes its downward way through the perineum, then ascends along the middle of the spinal column, and reaches Fengfu(DU16) at the back of the neck where it enters the brain. It continues to ascend from Fengfu(DU16), along the midline of the head and passing the vertex, forehead, columella of the nose and the upper lip, then to Yinjiao(DU28).

The branches from this channel connect with the kidney and travel through the heart.

(2) Points of the Du Meridian, DU

Changqiang(DU1)

Location: Below the tip of the coccyx, at the midpoint of the line connecting the tip of the coccyx and anus.

Indications: Diarrhea, hematochezia, hemorrhoid, prolapse of rectum, constipation, pain along the spinal column, lumbago, epilepsy.

Yaoshu(DU2)

Location: On the sacrum and on the posterior midline, just at the sacral hiatus.

Indications: Irregular menstruation, aching pain and stiffness of the back and low back, hemorrhoid, flaccidity of the lower extremities, epilepsy.

Yaoyangguan(DU3)

Location: On the low back and on the posterior midline, in the depression below the spinous process of the 4th lumbar vertebra.

Indications: Irregular menstruation, emission, impotency, lumbosacral pain, flaccidity of the lower extremities.

Mingmen(DU4)

Location: On the low back and on the posterior midline, in the depression below the spinous process of the 2nd lumbar vertebra.

Indications: Stiffness of the spinal column, lumbago, impotency, emission, irregular menstruation, diarrhea due to indigestion, abnormal vaginal discharge.

Xuanshu(DU5)

Location: On the low back and on the posterior midline, in the depression below the spinous process of the 1st lumbar vertebra.

Indications: Stiffness of the back and low back, diarrhea due to indigestion.

Jizhong(DU6)

Location: On the low back and on the posterior midline, in the depression below the spinous process of the 11th thoracic vertebra.

Indications: Epigastric pain, diarrhea, jaundice, epilepsy, stiffness of the back and low back.

Zhongshu(DU7)

Location: On the low back and on the posterior midline, in the depression below the spinous process of the 10th thoracic vertebra.

Indications: Epigastric pain, lumbago, stiffness of the back.

Jinsuo(DU8)

Location: On the low back and on the posterior midline, in the depression below the spinous process of the 9th thoracic vertebra.

Indications: Epilepsy, stiffness of the back, stomachache.

Zhiyang(DU9)

Location: On the low back and on the posterior midline, in the depression below the spinous process of the 7th thoracic vertebra.

Indications: Jaundice, cough with dyspnea, stiffness of the back, chest pain and backache.

Lingtai(DU10)

Location: On the low back and on the posterior midline, in the depression below the spinous process of the 6th thoracic vertebra.

Indications: Cough with dyspnea, furuncle, stiffness of the back and low back.

Shendao(DU11)

Location: On the low back and on the posterior midline, in the depression below the spinous process of the 5th thoracic vertebra.

Indications: Amnesia, palpitation, stiffness of the back and low back, cough, precordial pain.

Shenzhu(DU12)

Location: On the low back and on the posterior midline, in the depression below the spinous process of the 3rd thoracic vertebra.

Indications: Cough with dyspnea, epilepsy, stiffness of the back and low back.

Taodao(DU13)

Location: On the low back and on the posterior midline, in the depression below the spinous process of the 1st thoracic vertebra

Indications: Stiffness of back, headache, marlaria, fever.

Dazhui(DU14)

Location: On the posterior midline, in the depression below the spinous process of the 7th cervical vertebra

Indications: Headache complicated with stiffness of nape and back, marlaria, fever, epilepsy, hectic fever, cough with dyspnea, common cough.

Yamen(DU15)

Location: On the nape, 1.5 cun directly above the midpoint of the posterior hairline, below the 1st cervical vertebra.

Indications: Manic-depressive psychosis, epilepsy, deaf-mutism, sudden loss of voice, apoplexy, stiff tongue, pain in the occipital region, stiffness of nape, epistaxis.

Puncture perpendicularly 0.5-0.8 cun. Deep stabbing or puncturing upwards prohibited. The angle and depth should be controlled accurately.

Fengfu(DU16)

Location: On the nape, 1 cun directly above the midpoint of the posterior hairline, directly below the external occipital protuberance, in the depression between the trapezius muscle of both sides.

Indications: Headache, neck rigidity, blurred vision, epistaxis, sore throat, post-apoplectic aphasia, manic-depressive disorders, epilepsy.

Puncture perpendicularly 0.5-1 cun. Deep insertion prohibited.

Naohu(DU17)

Location: On the head, 2.5 cun above the midpoint of the posterior hairline, 1.5 cun above Fengfu(DU16), in the depression on the upper border of the external occipital protuberance.

Indications: Epilepsy, dizziness, stiffness of the nape and neck.

Qiangjian (DU18)

Location: On the head, 4 cun above the midpoint of the posterior hairline, 1.5 cun above Naohu (DU17).

Indications: Headache, stiffness of nape, giddiness, manic-depressive psychosis.

Houding (DU19)

Location: On the head, 5.5 cun above the midpoint of the posterior hairline, 3 cun above Naohu (DU17).

Indications: Headache, dizziness, manic-depressive psychosis, epilepsy.

Baihui (DU20)

Location: On the head, 5 cun directly above the midpoint of the anterior hairline, at the midpoint of the line connecting the apexes of both ears.

Indications: Headache, blurred vision, nasal obstruction, tinnitus, post-apoplectic aphasia, mental disorders, epilepsy, prolapse of the rectum, insomnia.

Qianding (DU21)

Location: On the head, 3.5 cun directly above the midpoint of the anterior hairline and 1.5 cun anterior to Baihui (DU20).

Indications: Epilepsy, dizziness and lightheadedness, pain in the vertex, rhinorrhea with turbid discharge.

Xinhui (DU22)

Location: On the head, 2 cun directly above the midpoint of the anterior hairline and 3 cun anterior to Baihui (DU20).

Indications: Headache, vertigo, rhinorrhea with turbid discharge.

Shangxing (DU23)

Location: On the head, 1 cun directly above the midpoint of the anterior hairline.

Indications: Headache, ophthalmalgia, rhinorrhea, epistaxis, malaria, febrile diseases, manic-depressive disorders, epilepsy.

Shenting (DU24)

Location: On the head, 0.5 cun directly above the midpoint of the anterior hairline.

Indications: Epilepsy, palpitation, insomnia, headache, dizziness, rhinorrhea with turbid discharge.

Suliao (DU25)

Location: On the face, at the centre of the nose apex.

Indications: Nasal obstruction, epistaxis, rhinorrhea, dyspnea, loss of consciousness, convulsion, asphyxia neonatorum.

Shuigou (DU26)

Location: On the face, at the junction of the upper third and middle third of the philtrum.

Indications: Manic-depressive disorders, epilepsy, infantile convulsion, coma, trismus, puffiness of the face, deviation of the mouth and eye, pain and stiffness of the lower back.

Duiduan (DU27)

Location: On the face, on the labial tubercle of the upper lip, on the vermilion border between the philtrum and upper lip.

Indications: Manic-depressive psychosis, hemiparalysis of face complicate with twitching and stiffness of the lips, gingivitis.

Yinjiao (DU28)

Location: Inside the upper lip, at the junction of the labial frenum and upper gum.

Indications: Manic-depressive psychosis, gingivitis, rhinorrhea with turbid discharge.

14. The Ren Channel

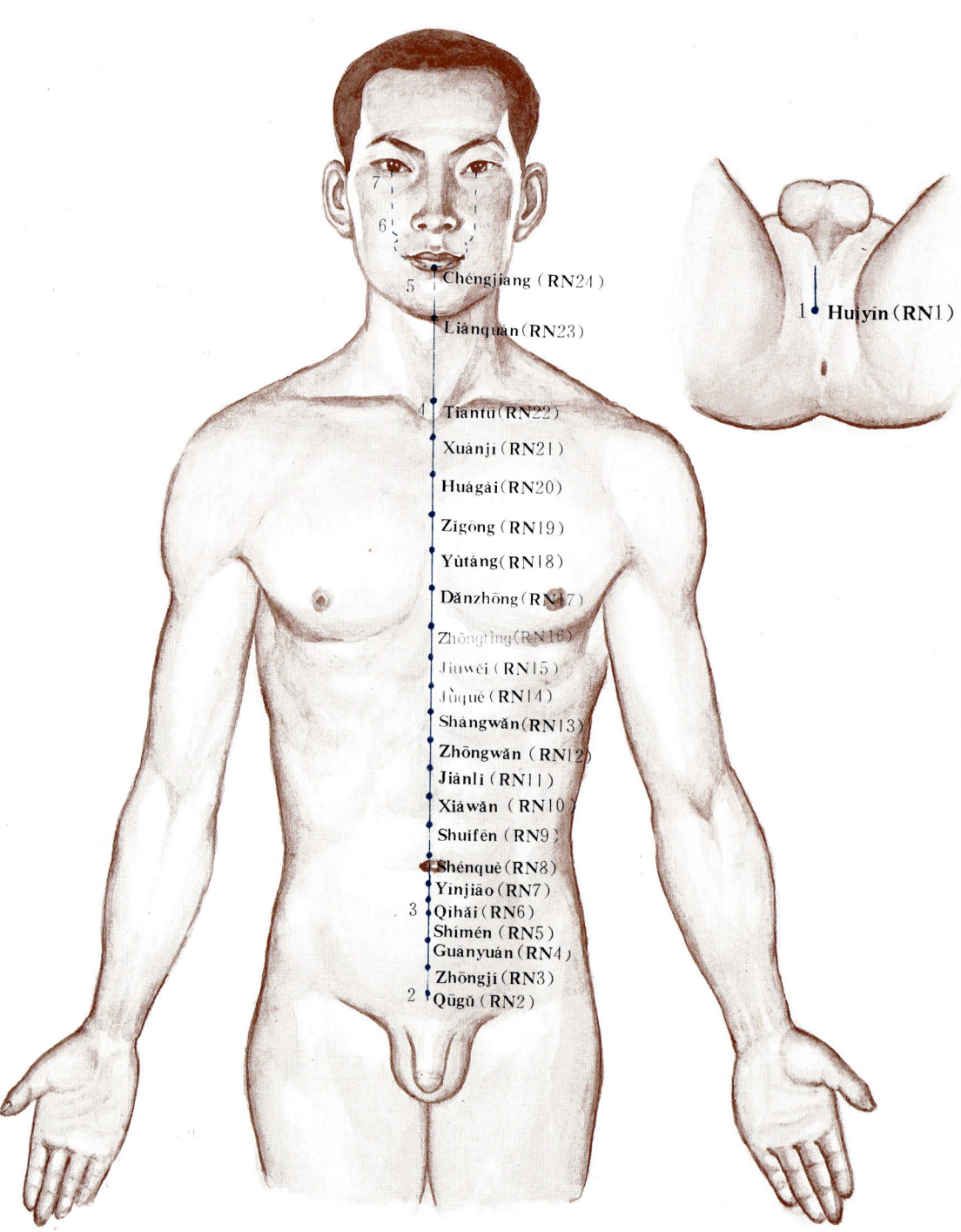

Fig. 16

The word "Ren" in Chinese means "take charge". The Ren Channel runs along the midline of the venter, meets with the three Yin Channels of the Hand and Foot as well as the Yinwei Channel many times in its course, and takes charge of all the yin channels of the whole body, so it is also named "the sea of all the yin channels". In addition, as the Ren Channel is related to pregnancy, there is a way of saying it, "the Ren Channel is in charge of pregnancy".

(1) Course

This channel originates in the uterus, and makes its downward way through the perineum, across the pubisure part, along the midline of the abdomen and the chest, through the throat to the mandible where it turns round the lips and up to Yinjiao(DU28). Via the face, two branches of the channel ascend to the regions below the orbits of the eyes.

(2) Points of the Ren Meridian, RN

Huiyin(RN1)

Location: On the perineum, at the midpoint between the posterior border of the scrotum and anus in male, and between the posterior commissure of the large labia and anus in female.

Indications: Pruritus vulvae, dysuria, hemorrhoid, emission, enuresis, irregular menstruation, manic-depressive psychosis.

Qugu(RN2)

Location: On the lower abdomen and on the anterior midline, at the midpoint of the upper border of the pubic symphysis.

Indications: Dribbling urination, retention of urine, enuresis, emission, impotency, abnormal vaginal discharge, irregular menstruation, dysmenorrhea, hernia.

Zhongji(RN3)

Location: On the lower abdomen and on the anterior midline, 4 cun below the centre of the umbilicus.

Indications: Enuresis, emission, impotency, hernia, metrorrhagia and metrostaxis, dysmenorrhea, irregular menstruation, abnormal vaginal discharge, frequency of micturition, retention of urine, pain in the lower abdomen, prolapse of uterus, pruritus vulvae.

Guanyuan(RN4)

Location: On the lower abdomen and on the anterior midline, 3 cun below the centre of the umbilicus.

Indications: Enuresis, nocturnal emission, frequency of micturition, retention of urination, hernia, irregular menstruation, abnormal vaginal discharge, dysmenor hea, metrorrhagia and metrostaxis, postpartum hemorrhage, pain in the lower abdomen, indigestion, diarrhea, prolapse of rectum, apoplexy marked by prostration syndrome.

Shimen(RN5)

Location: On the lower abdomen and on the anterior midline, 2 cun below the centre of the umbilicus.

Indications: Abdominal pain, diarrhea, edema, hernia, anuresis, enuresis, amenorrhea, abnormal vaginal discharge, metrorrhagia and metrostaxis, postpartum hemorrhage.

Qihai(RN6)

Location: On the lower abdomen and on the anterior midline, 1.5 cun below the centre of the umbilicus.

Indications: Pain in the lower abdomen, enuresis, emission, impotency, hernia, edema, diarrhea, dysentery, metrorrhagia and metrostaxis, irregular menstruation, dysmenorrhea, amenorrhea, morbid leukorrhee, postpartum hemorrhage, constipation, apoplexy presented by prostration syndrome.

Yinjiao(RN7)

Location: On the lower abdomen and on the anterior midline, 1 cun below the centre of the umbilicus.

Indications: Distention of the abdomen, edema, hernia, irregular menstruation, metrorrhagia and metrostaxis, morbid leukorrhage, pruritus vulvae, postpartum hemorrhage, pain around the umbilicus.

Shenque(RN8)

Location: On the middle abdomen and at the centre of the umbilicus.

Indications: Abdominal pain, borborygmus, apoplexy characterized by prostration syndrome, prolapse of the rectum, intractable diarrhea.

Puncture prohibited. Moxibustion with ginger or salt is more often used, apply 3-5 moxa cones or 10-30 minutes' moxibustion.

Shuifen(RN9)

Location: On the upper abdomen and on the anterior midline, 1 cun above the centre of the umbilicus.

Indications: Abdominal pain accompanied with borborygmus, edema, dysuria, diarrhea.

Xiawan(RN10)

Location: On the upper abdomen and on the anterior midline, 2 cun above the centre of the umbilicus.

Indications: Pain in the epigastric region and lower abdomen, borborygmus, indigestion, vomiting and diarrhea.

Jianli(RN11)

Location: On the upper abdomen and on the anterior midline, 3 cun above the centre of the umbilicus.

Indications: Stomachache, vomiting, distention of the abdomen, borborygmus, edema, anorexia.

Zhongwan(RN12)

Location: On the upper abdomen and on the anterior midline, 4 cun above the centre of the umbilicus.

Indications: Gastric pain, abdominal distention, borborygmus, vomiting with nausea, diarrhea, dysentery, jaundice, indigestion, insomnia.

Shangwan(RN13)

Location: On the upper abdomen and on the anterior midline, 5 cun above the centre of the umbilicus.

Indications: Stomachache, distention of the abdomen, nausea and vomiting, epilepsy, insomnia.

Juque(RN14)

Location: On the upper abdomen and on the anterior midline, 6 cun above the centre of the umbilicus.

Indications: Precordial pain, regurgitation of acid and food, dysphgia, vomiting, manic-depressive psychosis, epilepsy, palpitation.

Jiuwei(RN15)

Location: On the upper abdomen and on the anterior midline, 1 cun below the xiphisternal synchondrosis.

Indications: Precordial pain, regurgitation, manic-depressive psychosis, epilepsy.

Zhongting(RN16)

Location: On the chest and on the anterior midline, on the level of the 5th intercostal space, on the xiphisternal synchondrosis.

Indications: Distention of the chest and hypochondriac region, dysphagia, regurgitation.

Danzhong(RN17)

Location: On the chest and on the anterior midline, on the level of the 4th intercostal space, at the midpoint of the line connecting both nipples.

Indications: Dyspnea, hiccup, dysphagia, chest pain, palpitation, insufficient lactation.

Yutang(RN18)
Location: On the chest and on the anterior midline, on the level of the 3rd intercostal space.
Indications: Chest pain, cough with dyspnea, vomiting.

Zigong(RN19)
Location: On the chest and on the anterior midline, on the level of the 2nd intercostal space.
Indications: Chest pain, cough with dyspnea.

Huagai(RN20)
Location: On the chest and on the anterior midline, on the level of the 1st intercostal space.
Indications: Distending pain in the chest and hypochondriac region, cough with dyspnea.

Xuanji(RN21)
Location: On the chest and on the anterior midline, 1 cun below Tiantu(RN22).
Indications: Chest pain, cough with dyspnea.

Tiantu(RN22)
Location: On the neck and on the anterior midline, at the centre of the suprasternal fossa.
Indications: Asthma, cough, sore-throat, dry throat, hiccup, sudden loss of voice, dysphagia, goiter.

Lianquan(RN23)
Location: On the neck and on the anterior midline, above the laryngeal protuberance, in the depression above the upper border of the hyoid bone.
Indications: Swelling and pain of the subglossal region, salivation with flaccid tongue, stiffness of tongue due to apoplexy, sudden hoarseness of voice, difficulty in swallowing.

Chengjiang(RN24)
Location: On the face, in the depression at the midpoint of the mentolabial sulcus.
Indications: Edema of the face, swelling of the gums, salivation, manic-depress ivepsychosis, hemiparalysis of face.

Section 3 Location of The Extra Points

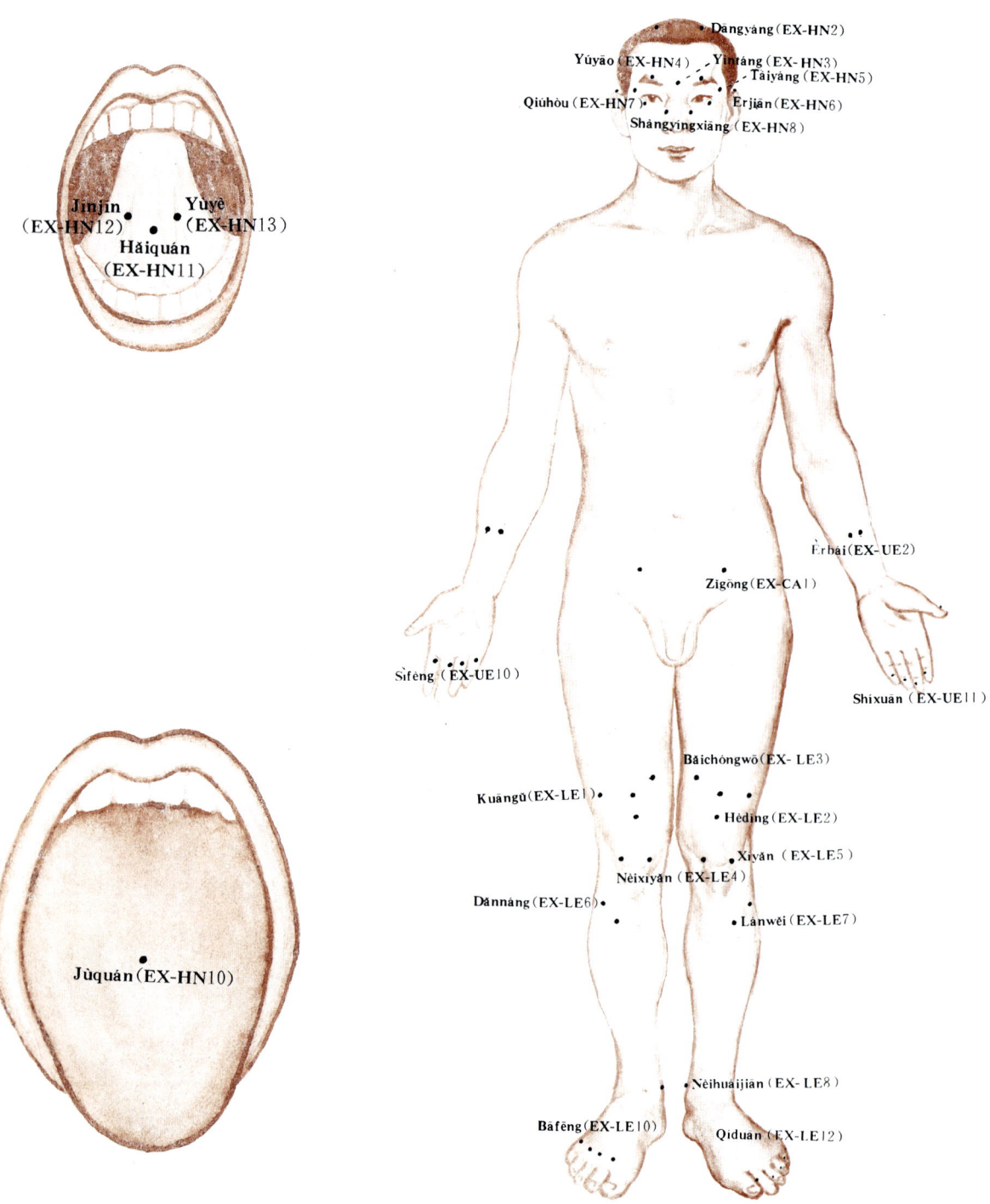

Fig. 17

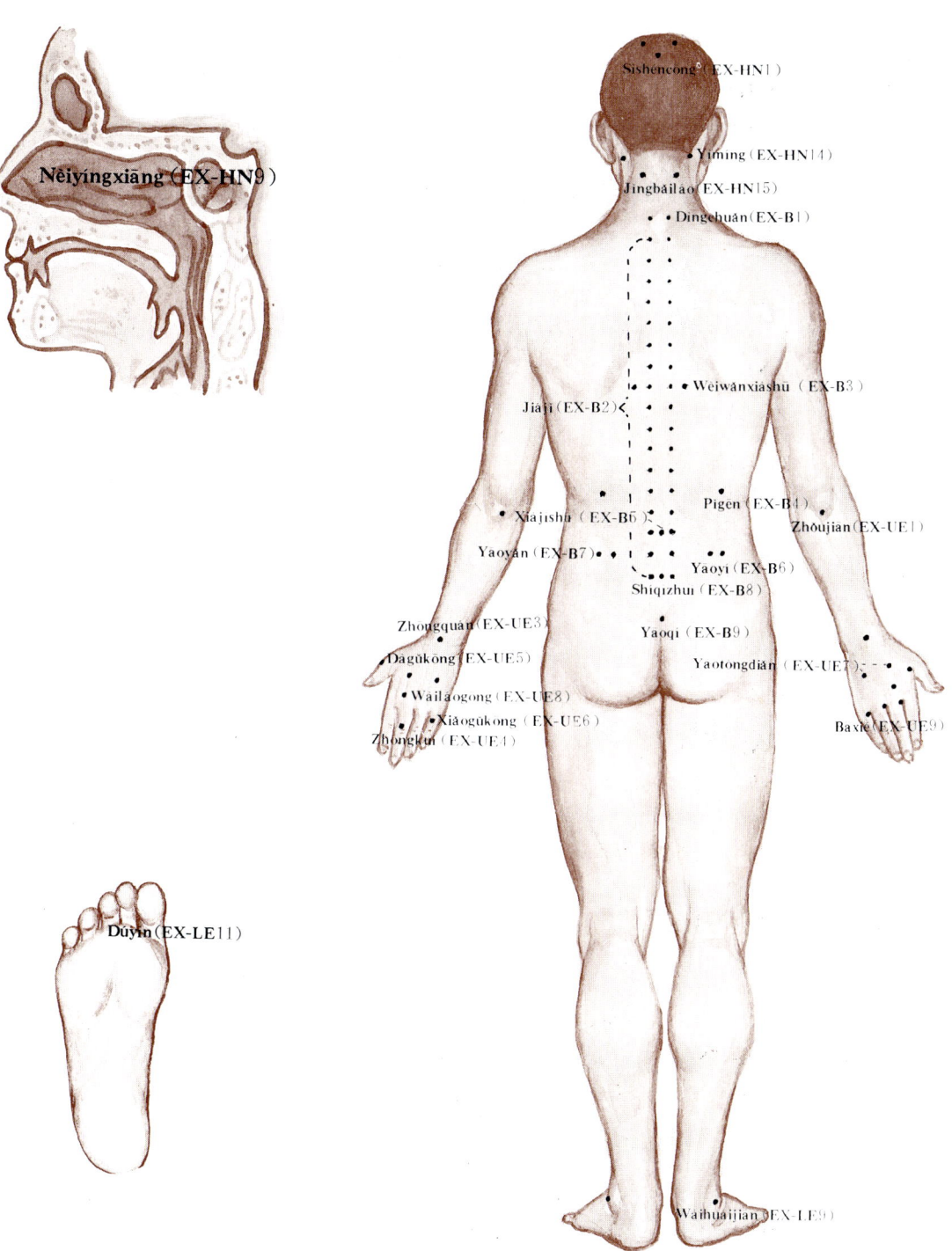

Fig. 18

1. Points of the Head and Neck, EX-HN

(Sishencong)EX-HN1
Location: Four points on the vertex of the head, 1 cun anterior, posterior and lateral to Baihui(DU20).
Indications: Headache, dizziness, insomnia, amnesia, epilepsy.

Dangyang(EX-HN2)
Location: At the frontal part of the head, directly above the pupil, 1 cun above the pupil, 1 cun above the anterior hairline.
Indications: Dizziness, ophthalmalgia, stuffy nose, common cough, headache, conjunctivitis, apoplectic stroke.

Yintang(EX-HN3)
Location: On the forehead, at the midpoint between the eyebrows.
Indications: Headache, heaviness sensation of the head, epistaxis, rhinorrhea with discharge, infantile convulsion, pain in the forehead, insomnia.

Yuyao(EX-HN4)
Location: On the forehead, at the midpoint between the eyebrows.
Indications: Pain in the supraorbital bone, twitching of eyelid(s), blepharoptosis, nebula, conjunctival congestion and swelling of the eye(s).

Taiyang(EX-HN5)
Location: At the temporal part of the head, between the lateral end of the eyebrow and the outer canthus, in the depression one finger breadth behind them.
Indications: Headache, ophthalmic disorders, hemiparalysis of face.

Erjian(EX-HN6)
Location: Above the apex of the ear auricle, at the tip of the auricle when the ear is folded forward.
Indications: Conjunctival congestion and swelling of the eye(s), fever, nebula.

Qiuhou(EX-HN7)
Location: On the face, at the junction of the lateral fourth and medial three fourths of the infraorbital margin.
Indications: Ophthalmic disorders.
Push gently the eyeball upward and then puncture perpendicularly and slowly 0.5-1.2 cun along the infraorbital margin. Strong twirling or lifting and thrusting the needle is not advisable.

Shangyingxiang(EX-HN8)
Location: On the face, at the junction of the alar cartilage of the nose and the nasal concha, near the upper end of the nasolabial groove.
Indications: rhinorrhea with turbid discharge, stuffy nose, boil of nose.

Neiyingxiang(EX-HN9)
Location: In the nostril, at the junction between the mucosa of the alar cartilage of the nose and the nasal concha.
Indications: Conjunctival congestion and swelling of the eye(s), rhinopathy, inflammation of the throat, fever, heatstroke, dizziness.
Prick to cause bleeding. Prohibited on cases with hemorrhagic diathesis.

Juquan(EX-HN10)
Location: In the mouth, at the midpoint of the dorsal midline of the tongue.
Indications: Stiff tongue, flaccid tongue with aphasia, diabetes, asthma, cough, hypogeusesthesia.

Haiquan(EX-HN11)
Location: In the mouth, at the midpoint of the frenulum of the tongue.
Indications: Diabetes, double tongue with swelling pain, laryngemphraxis, vomiting, diarrhea.

Jinjin(EX-HN12)
Location: In the mouth, on the vein in the left side of the frenulum of the tongue.
Indications: Swelling of tongue, intractable vomiting, stiff tongue.

Yuye(EX-HN13)
Location: In the mouth, on the vein in the right side of the frenulum of the tongue.
Indications: Swelling of tongue, intractable vomiting, stiff tongue.

Yiming(EX-HN14)
Location: On the nape, 1 cun posterior to Yifeng(SJ17).
Indications: Ophthalmic disorders, tinnitus, insomnia.

Jingbailao(EX-HN15)
Location: On the nape, 2 cun directly above Dazhui(DU14) and 1 cun lateral to the posterior midline.
Indications: Scrofula, cough, asthma, pertussis, stiffneck.

2. Points of the Chest and Abdomen, EX-CA

Zigong(EX-CA1)
Location: On the lower abdomen, 4 cun below the centre of the umbilicus and 3 cun lateral to Zhongji(RN3).
Indications: Prolapse of uterus, irregular menstruation.

(3) Points of Back, EX-B

Dingchuan(EX-B1)
Location: On the back, below the spinous process of the 7th cervical vertebra, 0.5 cun lateral to the posterior midline.
Indications: Asthmna, cough, stiffness of the nape, pain in the shoulder and back, rubella.

Jiaji(EX-B2)
Location: On the back and low back, 17 points on each side, below the spinous processes from the 1st thoracic to the 5th lumbar vertebrae, 0.5 cun lateral to the posterior midline.
Indications: Points on the upper portion of the chest can be used to treat diseases of the heart and lung and diseases in the upper limbs; points on the lower portion of the chest, gastrointestinal diseases; points on the lumbar region, diseases in the lumbar and abdominal regions and disorders in the lower extremities.

Weiwanxiashu(EX-B3)
Location: On the back, below the spinous process of the 8th thoracic vertebra, 1.5 cun lateral to the posterior midline.
Indications: Diabetes, vomiting, abdominal pain, pain in the chest and hypochondriac region.

Pigen(EX-B4)
Location: On the low back, below the spinous process of the 1st lumbar vertebra, 3.5 cun lateral to the posterior

midline.

Indications: Mass in the abdomen.

Xiajishu(EX-B5)

Location: On the midline of the low back, below the spinous process of the third lumbar vertebra.

Indications: Lumbago, abdominal pain, diarrhea, dysuria, enuresis, aching pain in the lower extremities.

Yaoyi(EX-B6)

Location: On the low back, below the spinous process of the 4th lumbar vertebra, 3 cun lateral to the posterior midline.

Indications: Lumbago, frequency of micturition, irregular menstruation.

Yaoyan(EX-B7)

Location: On the low back, below the spinous process of the 4th lumbar vertebra, in the depression 3.5 cun lateral to the posterior midline.

Indications: Lumbago, frequency of micturition, irregular menstruation, weakness with weight loss.

Shiqizhui(EX-B8)

Location: On the low back and on the posterior midline, below the spinous process of the 5th lumbar vertebra.

Indications: Lumbago, pain in the lower extremities, flaccidity of the lower extremity(ies), irregular menstruation, dysmenorrhea.

Yaoqi(EX-B9)

Location: On the low back, 2 cun directly above the tip of the coccyx, in the depression between the sacral horns.

Indications: Epilepsy, headache, insomnia, constipation.

4. Points of Upper Extremities, EX-UE

Zhoujian(EX-UE1)

Location: On the posterior side of the elbow, at the tip of the olecranon when the elbow is flexed.

Indications: Scrofula.

Erbai(EX-UE2)

Location: Two points on the palmar side of each forearm, 4 cun proximal to the crease of the wrist, on each side of the tendon of the radial flexor muscle of the wrist.

Indications: Pain due to hemorrhoid, prolapse of rectum.

Zhongquan(EX-UE3)

Location: On the dorsal crease of the wrist, in the depression on the radial side of the tendon of the common extensor muscle of the fingers.

Indications: Distention of the chest and hypochondriac region, cough with dyspnea, epigastric pain, precordial pain, hemoptysis, nebula, feverish sensation in the palm(s), distending pain in the abdomen.

Zhongkui(EX-UE4)

Location: On the dorsal crease of the middle finger, at the centre of the proximal interphalangeal joint.

Indications: Nausea, vomiting, hiccup.

Dagukong(EX-UE5)

Location: On the dorsal crease of the thumb, at the centre of the interphalangeal joint.

Indications: Ophthalmalgia, nebula, optic atrophy, vomiting with diarrhea, epistaxis.

Xiaogukong(EX-UE6)
Location: On the dorsal crease of the little finger, at the centre of the proximal interphalangeal joint.

Indications: Conjunctival congestion and swelling pain in the eye(s), nebula, sore-throat, pain in the phalangeal joint of hand.

Yaotongdian(EX-UE7)
Location: Two points on the dorsum of each hand, between the 1st and 2nd between the 3rd and 4th metacarpal bones, and at the midpoint between the dorsal crease of the wrist and the metacarpophalangeal joint.

Indications: Lumbar sprain.

Wailaogong(EX-UE8)
Location: On the dorsum of the hand, between the 2nd and 3rd metacarpal bones, and 0.5 cun proximal to the metacarpophalangeal joint.

Indications: Stiffneck, pain in the shoulder and upper arm.

Baxie(EX-UE9)
Location: Four points on the dorsum of each hand, at the junction of the red and white skin proximal to the margin of the webs between each two of the five fingers of a hand.

Indications: Fever complicated with dysphoria, numbness of the finger(s), contraction of the hand and forearm, swelling of the dorsum of hand.

Sifeng(EX-UE10)
Location: Four points on each hand, on the palmar side of the 2nd to 5th fingers and at the centre of the proximal interphalangeal joints.

Indications: Infantile malnutrition, pertussis.

Shixuan(EX-UE11)
Location: Ten points on both hands, at the tips of the 10 fingers, 0.1 cun from the free margin of the nails.

Indications: Apoplexy, coma, epilepsy, high fever, tonsillitis, infantile convulsion, numbness of the finger tip(s).

5. Points of Lower Extremities, EX-LE

Kuangu(EX-LE1)
Location: Two points on each thigh, in the lower part of the anterior surface of the thigh, 1.5 cun lateral and medial to Liangqiu(ST34).

Indications: Pain in the lower extremities.

Heding(EX-LE2)
Location: Above the knee, in the depression of the midpoint of the upper border of the patella.

Indications: Pain in the lower extremities, weakness of the leg and foot, paralysis.

Baichongwo(EX-LE3)
Location: 3 cun above medial superior corner of the patella of the thigh with the knee flexed, i.e. 1 cun above Xuehai(SP10).

Indications: Rubella, eczema, malnutrition due to parasitic infestation.

Neixiyan(EX-LE4)
Location: In the depression medial to the patellar ligament when the knee is flexed.

Indications: Gonalgia.

Xiyan (EX-LE5)

Location: In the depression on both sides of the patellar ligament when the knee is flexed. The medial and lateral points are named "Neixiyan" and "Waixiyan" respectively.

Indications: Gonalgia, weakness of the lower extremities.

Dannang (EX-LE6)

Location: At the upper part of the lateral surface of the leg, 2 cun directly below the depression anterior and inferior to the head of the fibula [Yanglingquan (GB34)].

Indications: Acute or chronic cholecystitis, cholelithes, biliary ascariasis, flaccidity of the lower extremities.

Lanwei (EX-LE7)

Location: At the upper part of the anterior surface of the leg, 5 cun below Dubi (ST35), one finger breadth lateral to the anterior crest of the tibia.

Indications: Acute or chronic appendicitis, indigestion, paralysis of the lower extremities.

Neihuaijian (EX-LE8)

Location: On the medial side of the foot, at the tip of the medial malleolus.

Indications: Toothache, spasm of the medial portion of the foot.

Waihuaijian (EX-LE9)

Location: On the lateral side of the foot, at the tip of the lateral malleolus.

Indications: Spasm of the lateral portion of the foot, disturbance of lower legs due to pathogen of either cold or heat.

Bafeng (EX-LE10)

Location: Eight points on the instep of both feet, at the junction of the red and white skin proximal to the margin of the webs between each two neighbouring toes.

Indications: Beriberi, pain in the toe(s), swelling pain in the dorsum of foot.

Duyin (EX-LE11)

Location: On the plantar side of the 2nd toe, at the centre of the distal interphalangeal joint.

Indications: Sudden onset of precordial pain, pain in the chest and hypochondriac region, vomiting, hematemesis, stillborn fetus, retention of placenta, irregular menstruation, hernia.

Qiduan (EX-LE12)

Location: Ten points at the tips of the 10 toes of both feet, 0.1 cun from the free margin of each toenail.

Indications: Apoplexy, numbness of the toe(s), swelling pain in the dorsum of foot.

Chapter Two
The Eight Extra Channels

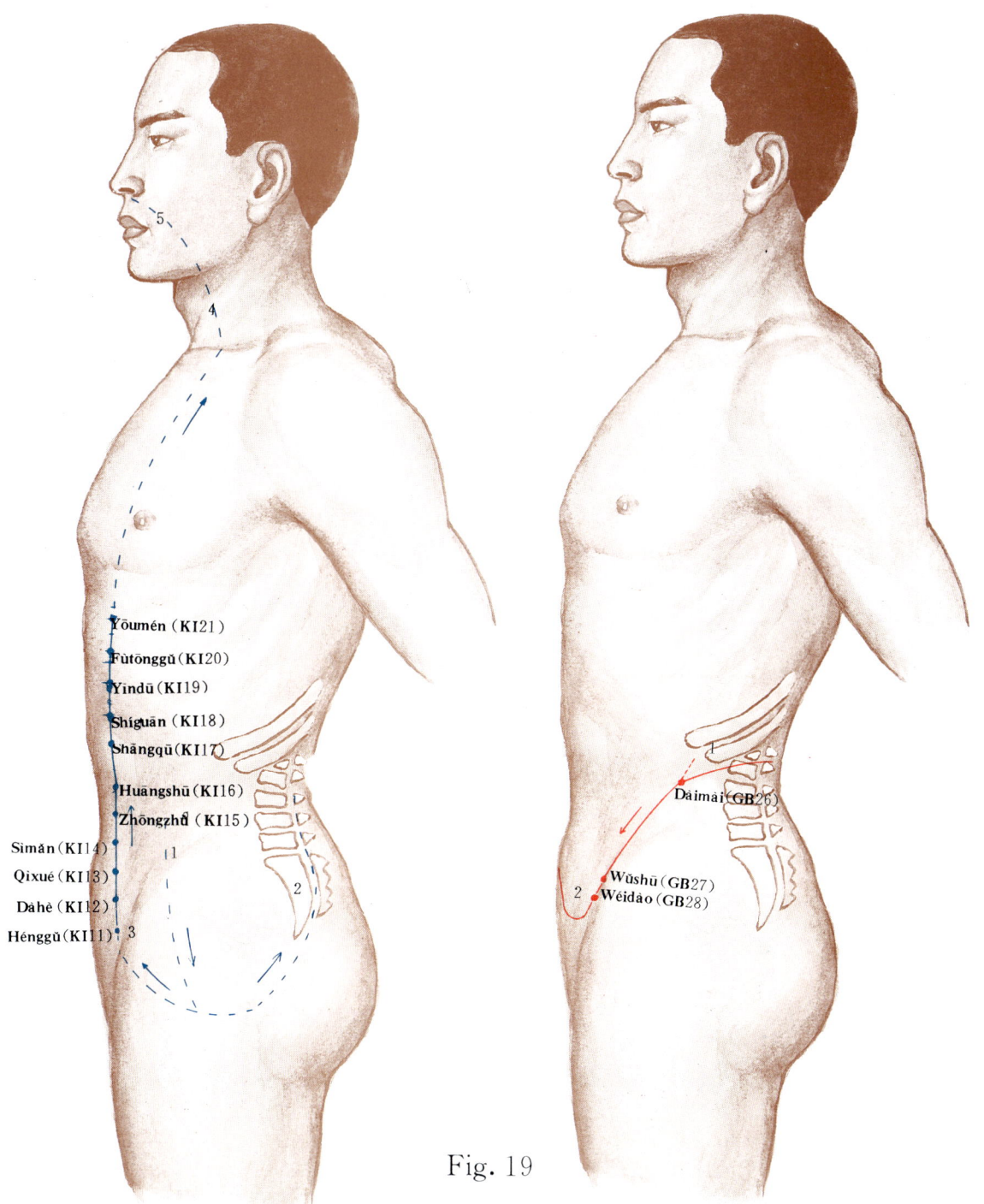

Fig. 19

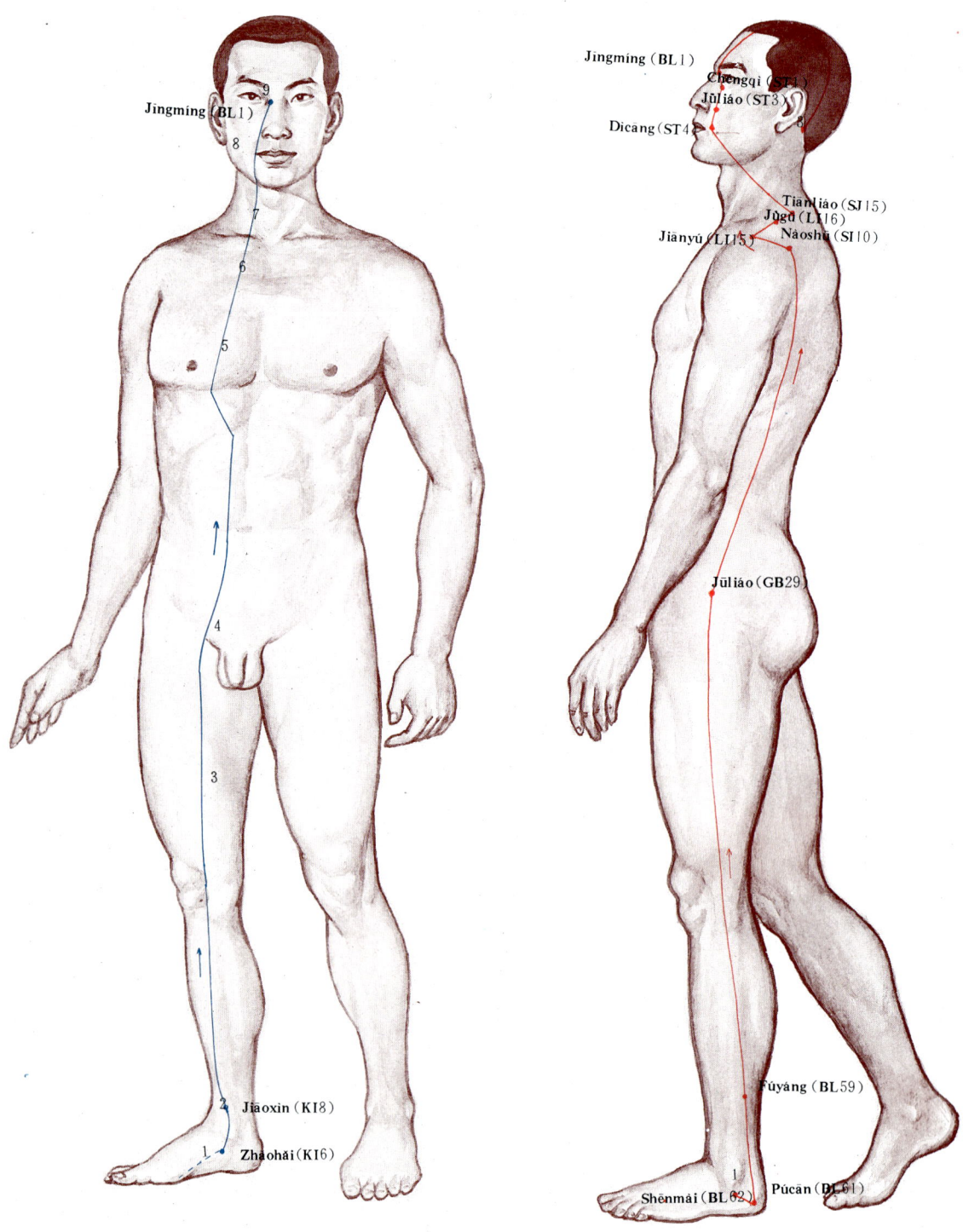

Fig. 20

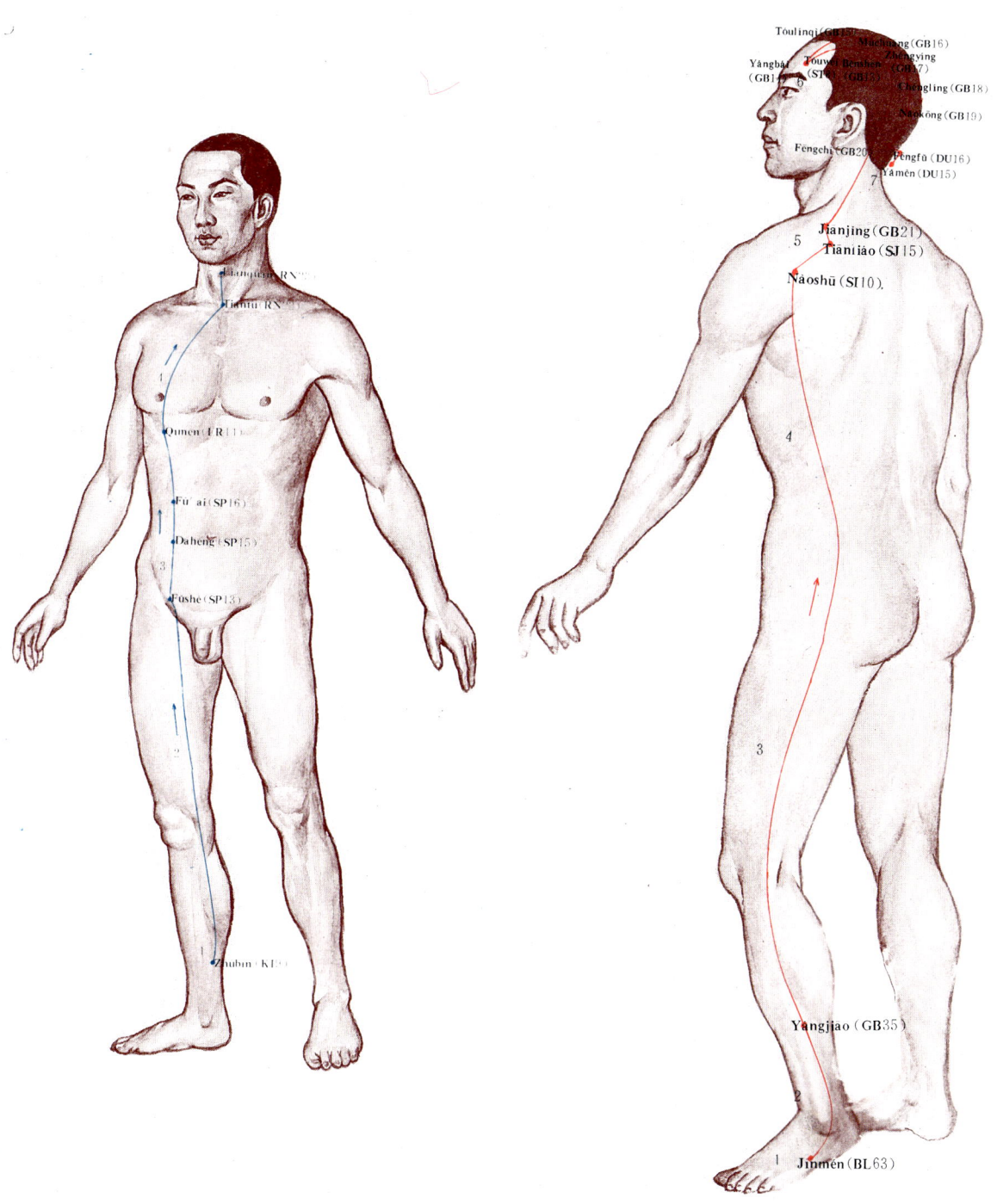

Fig. 21

"The Eight extra Channels" is general term for the Du, Ren, Chong, Dai, Yinqiao, Yangqiao, Yinwei and Yangwei Channels. They are called "the Eight Extra Channels" because their courses are not as regular as those of the above mentioned Twelve Channels, because they have no direct relationship with any of the internal organs, or exterior-interior coordination between them and because their total number is eight.

The Eight Extra Channels crisscross the regular twelve channels, and perform the functions of strengthening the ties between the channels and regulating the "qi" and blood inside the twelve regular channels. When the blood and qi inside the Twelve Channels are full and overflowing, the excess will be stored in the Eight Extra Channels. They are not only more closely related to the liver, kidney and other internal organs, but also to the uterus, brain, marrow and extra ordinary organs.

1. The Du Channel

2. The Ren Channel

The Du channel and Ren channel are to be described in Chapter 1.

2. The Ren Channel

3. The Chong Channel

The Chong Channel controls and regulates "qi" and blood inside the twelve regular channels, so it is named "the sea of the Twelve Channels" or "the sea of blood". This channel is closely related to the menses.

(1) Course

This channel originates in the uterus, descends and emerges at the perineum, then ascends through the spinal column. The superficial branch of the channel passes Point Qichong(ST30), meets with the Kidney Channel of Foot-Shaoyin, and runs along both sides of the abdomen, reaches the throat and finally goes round the lips.

(2) Pathological Symptoms

Menstrual disorder, uterine bleeding, sterility, hypogalactia, spitting blood, abnormal rising of qi, spasm in abdomen, etc..

4. The Dai Channel

The word "Dai" in Chinese means "a belt". The Dai Channel runs transversely round the waist like a belt. That is why it is termed the Dai Channel (the Belt Channel). It binds all the channels of the body, fixing and safeguarding the foetus and controlling the secretion of the leucorrhea.

(1) Course
This channel starts below the hypochondrium, descends obliquely to Point Daimai(GB26), then runs transversely round the waist.

2) Pathological Symptoms
Profuse leucorrhea, abortion, hysteroptosis, abdominal distention, soreness and debility of the waist, etc..

5. The Yinqiao Channel and the Yangqiao Channel

"Qiao" in Chinese means "nimble". The Yangqiao Channel can control the "yang" of the left and right sides of the whole body, while the Yinqiao Channel not only controls the "yin" of the left and right sides of the whole body, but also nourishes the eyes, controls the opening and closing of the eyelids as well as the motion of the lower limbs.

(1) Course
The Qiao Channels both originate in the region below the malleoli, but run separately along the left and right sides of the body.

The Yinqiao Channel ascends from Point Zhaohai(KI6) below the medial malleolus to the upper portion of the malleolus. Then it runs along the medio-posterior aspect of the lower limbs, straight to the external genitalia. From there it ascends further along the abdomen and chest into the supraclavicular fossa. Running along the throat, it passes in front of Point Renying(ST9) and the medial side of the zygomatic region, and reaches the inner canthus of the eye where the channel meets with the Taiyang Channels of both Hand and Foot as well as the Yangqiao Channel.

The Yangqiao Channel travel from Shenmai(BL62) below the external malleolus, up to the malleolus, through the posterior border of the fibula and the lateral side of the thigh, to the posterior aspect of the hypochondriac region. Via the posterior axillary fold, it winds its way through the shoulder and ascends along the neck to the corner of the mouth. Passing the side of the naris, it goes into the inner canthus where the channel communicates with the Taiyang Channels of the Hand and Foot as well as the Yinqiao Channel. From there it travels along the Urinary Bladder Channel of Foot-Taiyang to the forehead upward into the hairline, then goes behind the ear and meets with the GallBladder Channel of Foot-Shaoyang at Point Fengchi(GB20).

(2) Pathological Symptoms

Yinqiao disease is symptomatized by myasthenia of the lateral side of the limbs and myospasm of the medial side of the limbs, laryngalgia and somnolence. Yangqiao disease is symptomatized by myasthenia of the medial side of the limbs and myospasm of the lateral side of the limbs, insanity, insomnia and pain in the inner canthus.

6. The Yinwei Channel and the Yangwei Channel

"Wei" in Chinese means "maintain and communicate". The Yinwei Channel serves to maintain and communicate with all the yin channels of the body, while the Yangwei Channel serves all the yang channels.

(1) Course

The Yinwei Channel originates in the region where three yin channels cross at the medial aspect of the calf, ascends along the medial aspect of the lower extremities and reaches the abdomen to join the Spleen Channel of Foot-Taiyin. From there it runs upward to the hypochondrium to meet with the Liver Channel of Foot-Jueyin. Then it ascends along the chest to communicate with the Ren Channel at the neck.

The Yangwei Channel originates in the heel, exits from the external malleolus and ascends along the course of the Gall Bladder Channel of Foot-Shaoyang. It passes the lateral aspect of the lower extremity and posterolateral side of the trunk, ascends behind the axilla to the shoulder. From there it continues its travel through the neck towards the forehead, spreading over the sides of the head and the back of the neck and thus communicating with the Du Channel.

(2) Pathological Symptoms

Disturbance of the Yinwei Channel gives rise to the following symptoms: chest pain, stomachache and precordial pain. Disturbance of the Yangwei Channel causes symptoms such as alternate spells of chill and fever.

Chapter Three
Auricular Points

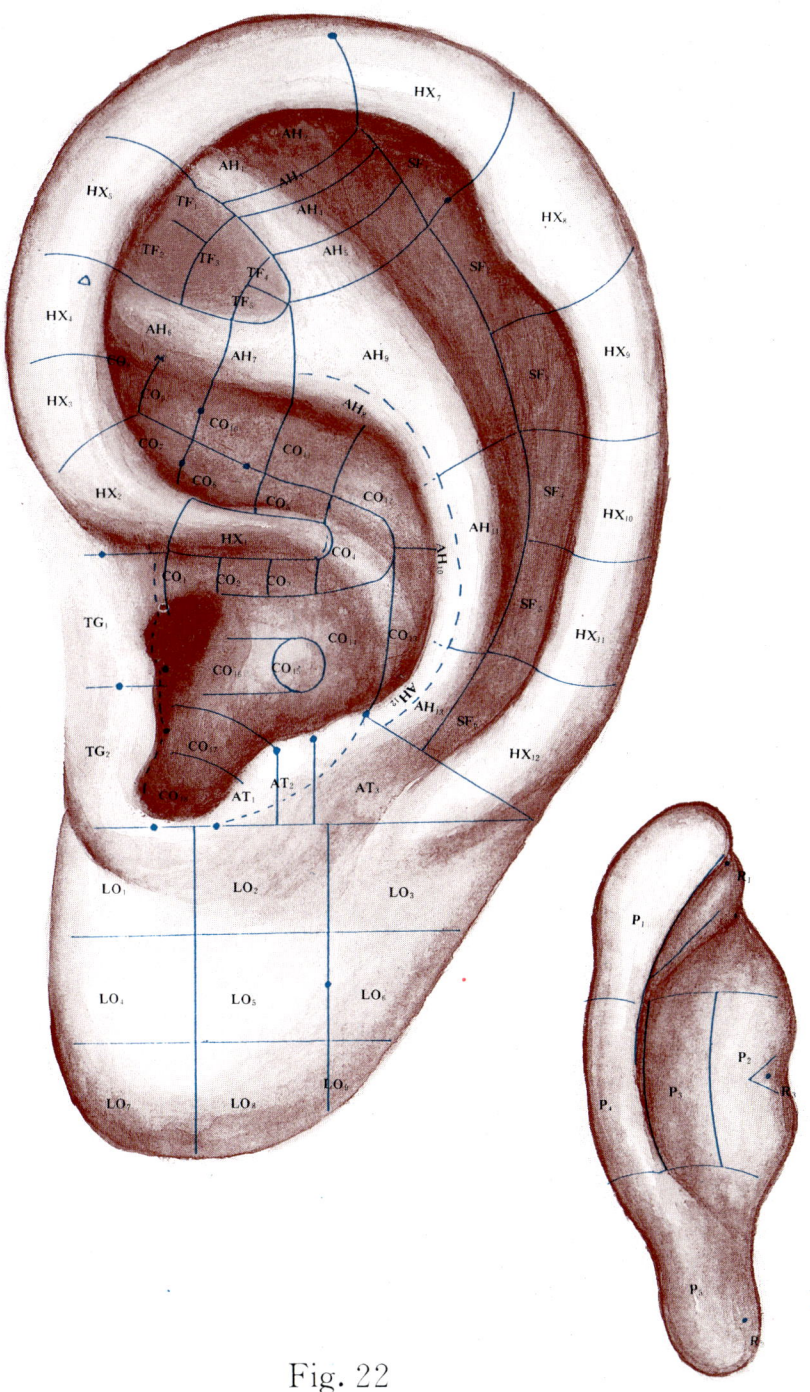

Fig. 22

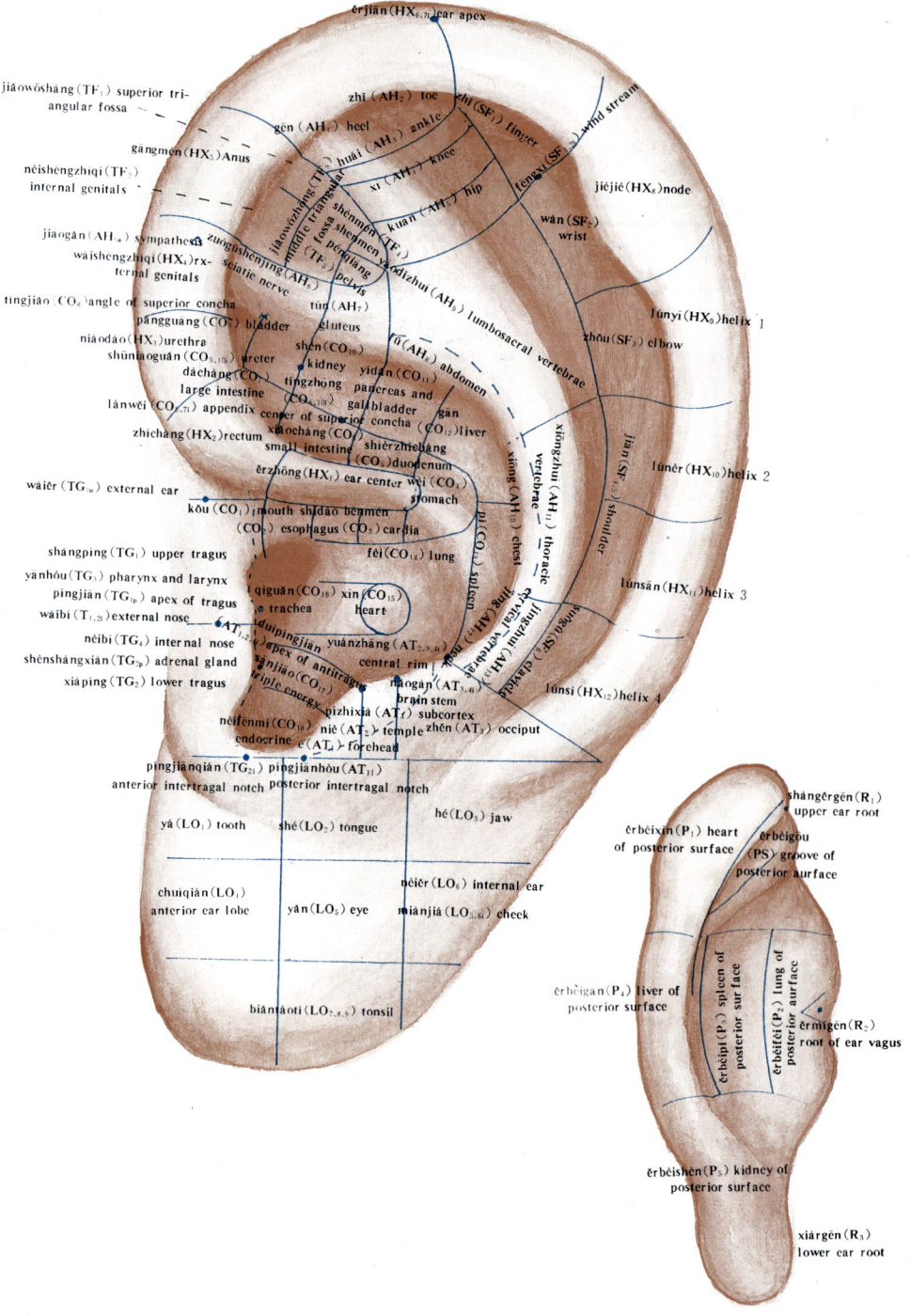

Fig. 23

1. Points on the Helix

Erzhong(HX1) ear centre
Location: On the helix crus.
Indications: Headache, tinnitus, deafness, hemoptysis, jaundice, urticaria, pruritus cutanea, infantile enuresis.

Zhichang(HX2) rectum
Location: On the helix anterior and superior to the spine of helix.
Indications: Diarrhea, constipation, prolapse of rectum, hemorrhoid.

Niaodao(HX3) urethra
Location: On the helix superior to Zhichang(HX2).
Indications: Enuresis, emergency of micturition, frequency of urination, urodynia, retention of urine, prostatitis.

Waishengzhiqi(HX4) external genitals
Location: On the helix anterior to the lower crus of helix.
Indications: Impotency, testitis, epididymitis, pruritus vulvae, urethritis, balanitis, lumbago and scelalgia.

Gangmen(HX5) anus
Location: On the helix anterior to the triangular fossa.
Indications: Hemorrhoid, anal fissure, prolapse of rectum, pruritus ani.

Erjian(HX6.7i) ear apex
Location: At the top of the helix, opposite to the posterior border of superior antihelix crus.
Indications: Fever, hypertension, acute conjunctivitis, hordeolum, neurosis, dermatosis.

Jiejie(HX8) node
Location: At the tubercle of the helix.
Indications: Dizziness, headache, hypertension, chronic hepatitis.

Lunyi(HX9) helix 1
Location: At the helix area from lower border of helix tubercle to the midpoint of lower border of ear lobe is divided into four equal parts, the points making the division are respectively HX9,10, 11, and 12. HX9 owns the first portion.
Indications: Fever, inflammation of the upper respiratory tract, tonsillitis, hypertension.

Luner(HX10) helix 2
Location: The second portion below HX9.
Indications: Fever, inflammation of the upper respiratory tract, tonsillitis.

Lunsan(HX11) helix 3
Location: On the third portion.
Indications: Fever, inflammation of the upper respiratory tract, tonsillitis.

(HX12) helix 4
Location: On the fourth portion, just below HX11.
Indications: Fever, inflammation of the upper respiratory tract, tonsillitis.

2. Points on the Scaphoid Fossa

Zhi(SF1) finger
Location: Divide the scapha into six portions from upward to downward, the first portion is SF1.

Indications: Pain and numbness of the fingers, paronychia, sprain of phalangeal joint of hand, Raynaud's disease, hyperhidrosis, dermatosis.

Wan(SF2) wrist
Location: The second portion of scapha.

Indications: Carpal pain, carpal arthritis, tenosynovitis.

Fengxi(SF3) wind stream
Location: Between SF1 and SF2 on capha.

Indications: Rhinallergosis, branchial asthma, urticaria, pruritus cutanea, irritable colon, allergic purpura.

Zhou(SF4) elbow
Location: The third portion of scapha.

Indications: Pain in the elbow, external humeral epicondylitis, cubital arthritis, sprain of elbow joint.

Jian(SF4,5) shoulder
Location: The area of the fourth and fifth portions of scapha.

Indications: Omalgia, scapulohumeral periarthritis, sprain of shoulder joint, pain in the upper arm.

Suogu(SF6) clavicle
Location: The sixth portion of scapha.

Indications: Scapulohumeral periarthritis, pulseless disease, pain in the shoulder and back.

3. Points on the Antihelix

Gen(AH1) heel
Location: At anterior upper corner of superior antihelix crus, near upper end of triangular fossa.

Indications: Painful heels, calcaneal spur.

Zhi(AH2) toe
Location: At posterior upper corner of superior antihelix crus, near the ear apex.

Indications: Paronychia, sprain of phalangeal joint of foot, cold injury, cold pain and numbness of toes, tinea pedis.

Huai(AH3) ankle
Location: Midway between AH1 and AH4.

Indications: Sprain of ankle, arthritis of ankle joint.

Xi(AH4) knee
Location: The middle 1/3 of superior antihelix crus.

Indications: Sprain of knee joint, gonitis, gonalgia.

Kuan(AH5) hip
Location: The lower 1/3 of superior antihelix crus.

Indications: Merocoxalgia, sciatica.

Zuogushenjing(AH6) sciatic nerve
Location: At the anterior 2/3 of inferior antihelix crus.

Indications: Sciatica.

Jiaogan(AH6a) sympathesis
Location: At the antihelix, on the junction between the termination of inferior antihelix crus and helix.

Indications: Gastritis, gastrospasm, palpitation, precordial pain, colic in the gallbladder, biliary calculi, calculus of kidney and urinary tract, hyperhidrosis, night sweat, asthma, thromboangiitis obliterans, phlebitis, aorto-arteritis, Raynaud's disease, seborrheic dermatitis, salivation.

Tun(AH7) gluteus
Location: At the posterior 1/3 of inferior antihelix crus.
Indications: Sciatica, fasciitis, sacral pain radiating to the buttock.

Fu(AH8) abdomen
Location: At the upper part of antihelix, the anterior 2/5 portion.
Indications: Abdominal pain, distention of the abdomen, diarrhea, constipation, lumbago, dysmenorrhea, pain due to uterine contraction.

Yaodizhui(AH9) lumbosacral vertebrae
Location: At the upper 2/5 of antihelix.
Indications: Lumbosacral pain, hyperosteogeny of lumbar vertebra, enuresis, sacroiliitis.

Xiong(AH10) chest
Location: At the middle part of the antihelix, at the anterior 2/5 portion.
Indications: Pain in the chest and hypochondriac region, chest distress, mastitis, pleurisy, costal chondritis, intercostal neuralgia, herpes zoster.

Xiongzhui(AH11) thoracic vertebrae
Location: At the middle 2/5 of antihelix.
Indications: Chest pain, distending pain in the breast prior to menstrual period, mastitis, hypogalactia.

Jing(AH12) neck
Location: The lower 2/5 portion of the anterior antihelix.
Indications: Stiffneck, cervical spondylopathy, torticollis, swelling pain in the neck and nape, cervical lymphadenitis, hyperthyroidism.

Jingzhui(AH13) cervical vertebrae
Location: At the antihelix the line from helix-tragic notch to the bifurcation between superior antihelix crus, the lower 1/5.
Indications: Stiffneck, cervical spondylopathy, cervical fibrositis.

4. Points on Triangular Fossa

Jiaowoshang(TF1) superior triangular fossa
Location: Anterior and superior of the triangular fossa.
Indications: Hypertensive diseases.

Neishengzhiqi(TF2) internal genitals
Location: In the anterior 1/3 of the triangular fossa.
Indications: Irregular menstruation, dysmenorrhea, dysfunctional uterine bleeding, amenorrhea, leukorrhea, endometrial inflammation.

Jiaowozhong(TF3) middle triangular fossa
Location: In the middle 1/3 of the triangular fossa.
Indications: Asthma.

Shenmen(TF4) shenmen
Location: In the triangular fossa, at the superior aspect of the bifurcating point between superior antihelix and inferior antihelix crus.

Indications: Insomnia, dreaminess, dizziness, cough with dyspnea, diarrhea.

Penqiang(TF5) pelvis

Location: In the triangular fossa, at the inferior aspect of the bifurcating point between superior antihelix crus and inferior antihelix crus.

Indications: Pelvic inflammation, prostatitis, impotency, pain in the lower abdominal region.

5. Points on the Tragus

Shangping(TG1) upper tragus

Location: Lateral margin of the tragus on the upper 1/2 portion.

Indications: Dizziness, otopathy, atrial fibrillation, paroxysmal tachycardia.

Xiaping(TG2) lower tragus

Location: Lateral margin of the tragus on the lower 1/2 portion.

Indications: Hyperthyroidism, diabetes, diabetes insipidus, adiposis.

Waier(TG1u) external ear

Location: On the superior border of the tragus, near the helix.

Indications: Inflammation of external auditory canal, otitis media, tinnitus, deafness, cold injury, rhinitis, nasal sinusitis, headache, dizziness, prosopalgia.

Pingjian(TG1p) apex of tragus

Location: At the tip of the prominence, superior to tragus.

Indications: Fever, toothache.

Waibi(TG1,2i) external nose

Location: At the anterior to the middle of the lateral aspect of tragus.

Indications: Rhinitis, nasal vestibulitis, furuncle, brandy nose, nasal acne.

Shenshangxian(TG2p) adrenal gland

Location: At the tip of the prominence, inferior to tragus.

Indications: Hypotension, dizziness due to streptomycin poisoning, cough with dyspnea, parotitis, rheumatism, malaria tertiana, collagen disease, anaphylaxis, dysfunctional uterine bleeding, hematochezia.

Yanhou(TG3) pharynx and larynx

Location: At the upper 1/2 portion of the inner surface of tragus.

Indications: Acute and chronic pharyngitis, tonsillitis, bronchitis, asthma, globus hystericus.

Neibi(TG4) internal nose

Location: At the lower 1/2 portion of the inner surface of tragus.

Indications: Cough, chronic rhinitis, nasal sinustis, epistaxis.

Pingjianxian(TG2l) anterior intertragal notch

Location: On the lower border of TG2.

Indications: Pseudomyopia, glaucoma, retinitis, iridocyclitis.

6. Points on the Antitragus

E(AT1) forehead

Location: At the anterior interior corner of lateral aspect of antitragus.

Indications: Dizziness, headache, insomnia, dreaminess, amnesia, hypertension, depression.

Pingjianhou(AT11) posterior intertragal notch
Location: On the lower border of antitragus.
Indications: Pseudomyopia, conjunctivitis, iridocyclitis, hordeolum.

Zhen(AT3) occiput
Location: At posterior superior corner of lateral aspect of antitragus.
Indications: Dizziness, headache, ametropia, asthma, vomiting, diarrhea, pruritus cutanea, epilepsy.

Pizhixia(AT4) subcortex
Location: At the interior aspect of antitragus.
Indications: Pseudomyopia, indigestion, ulcerative disease, distention of the abdomen, diarrhea, constipation, malaria, hypertension, arrhythmia, aorto-arteritis, thromboangiitis obliterans, phlebitis, Raynaud's disease, neurosis, schizophrenia.

Duipingjian(AT1,2,4i) apex of antitragus
Location: At the intersectio of AT1,2,4.
Indications: Bronchitis, asthma, parotitis, pruritus, cutanea, testitis, epididymitis.

Yuanzhong(AT2,3,4i) central rim
Location: At the intersectio of AT2,3,4.
Indications: Enuresis, hematochezia, irregular menstruation, dysfunctional uterine bleeding, amenorrhea, impotency, auditory vertigo, midget, diabetes insipidus, hypophysoma.

Naogan(AT3,4i) brain stem
Location: On the junction between the points AT3 and AT4.
Indications: Headache, dizziness, insomnia, schizophrenia, epilepsy, mild fever, bronchitis, deafness, tinnitus, allergic dermatitis.

7. Points on the Auricular Concha

Kou(CO1) mouth
Location: At the anterior 1/3, inferior to the helix crus.
Indications: Stomatitis, glossitis, periodontitis, pharyngitis, laryngitis, bronchitis, facial paralysis, disorders of temporomandibular joint, biliary calculi, cholecystitis, lumbago and scelalgia, insomnia, lassitude and fatigue.

Shidao(CO2) esophagus
Location: At the middle 1/3, inferior to the helix crus.
Indications: Dysphagia, esophagitis, esophagismus, chest distress, globus hystericus, hypopnea.

Benmen(CO3) cardia
Location: At the lower 1/3, inferior to the helix crus.
Indications: Spasm of cardia, nervous vomiting, nausea, discomfort in the chest.

Wei(CO4) stomach
Location: At the area where helix crus terminates.
Indications: Gastritis, gastric ulcer, gastric spasm or phrenospasm.

Shierzhichang(CO5) duodenum
Location: In the superior concha, posterior and superior to helix crus.
Indications: Duodenal bulbar ulcer, duodenitis, cholecystitis, calculi, pylorospasm.

Xiaochang(CO6) small intestine
Location: In the superior concha, superior and middle to helix crus.

Indications: Indigestion, abdominal pain, distention of the abdomen, diarrhea, constipation, oliguria with burning sensation during urination, stomatocace, pharyngitis, tachycardia, arrhythmia, hypogalactia.

Dachang(CO7) large intestine

Location: In the superior concha, anterior and superior to helix crus.

Indications: Distention of abdomen, diarrhea, constipation, rhinitis, pharyngitis, bronchitis, acne.

Lanwei(CO6,7i) appendix

Location: In the superior concha, between CO6 and CO7.

Indications: Appendicitis, diarrhea.

Tingjiao(CO8) angle of superior concha

Location: At anterior superior angle of superior concha.

Indications: Prostatitis, prostatic hyperplasia, sexual disorder, urethritis.

Pangguang(CO9) bladder

Location: In the superior concha between the points CO10 and CO8.

Indications: Enuresis, cystitis, retention of urine, lumbago, sciatica, occipital headache, insomnia.

Shen(CO10) kidney

Location: In the superior concha, inferior to bifurcating point between superior antihelix crus and inferior antihelix crus.

Indications: Lumbago, tinnitus, neurasthenia, pyelonephritis, asthma, enuresis, abnormal menstruation, spermatorrhea, prospermia.

Shuniaoguan(CO9,10i) ureter

Location: Between the points CO9 and CO10.

Indications: Ureterolithiasis and colic pain.

Yidan(CO11) pancreas and gallbladder

Location: In the superior concha, between the points CO12 and CO10.

Indications: Cholecystitis, cholelithiasis, biliary ascariasis, migraine, herpes, zoster, otitis media, tinnitus, poor hearing, acute pancreatitis.

Gan(CO12) liver

Location: At the posterior portion of superior concha.

Indications: Hypochondriac pain, dizziness, premenstrual tension, abnormal menstruation, climacteric syndrome, hypertension, pseudomyopia, simple glaucoma.

Tingzhong(CO6,10i) center of superior concha

Location: Between the points CO6 and CO10.

Indications: Abdominal pain and distention, biliary ascariasis, parotitis.

Pi(CO13) spleen

Location: Posterior and superior of the cavity of concha.

Indications: Abdominal distention, diarrhea, constipation, anorexia, dysfunctional uterine bleeding, leukorrhagia, auditory vertigo.

Xin(CO15) heart

Location: At the central point of cavity of concha.

Indications: Tachycardia, arrhythmia, angina pectoris, Takayasu's disease, neurasthenia, hysteria, ulcerations of mouth and tongue.

Qiguan(CO16) trachea

Location: In the inferior concha, between the opening of external auditory tract and point CO15.

Indications: Cough and asthma.

Fei(CO14) lung
Location: Around the centre of inferior concha.

Indications: Cough, asthma, fullness of chest, hoarseness of voice, acne, skin itching, verruca plana, flat wart, constipation, with drawal syndrome.

Sanjiao(CO17) triple energy
Location: At the fundus of inferior concha, superior to point CO18.

Indications: Constipation, abdominal distention, pain at the lateral side of the upper extremities.

Neifenmi(CO18) endocrine
Location: At the fundus of inferior concha, anterior and lower portion of the cavity of concha.

Indications: Dysmenorrhea, abnormal menstruation, climateric syndrome, acne, malaria.

8. Points on the Ear Lobe

Ya(LO1) tooth
Location: Upper portion on the anterior margin of lobe.

Indications: Toothache, periodontitis, hypotension.

She(LO2) tongue
Location: Middle and superior portion of lobe.

Indications: Glossitis, stomatitis.

He(LO3) jaw
Location: Upper portion on the posterior margin of lobe.

Indications: Toothache, temporomandibular arthritis.

Chuiqian(LO4) anterior ear lobe
Location: Middle portion, on the anterior margin of lobe.

Indications: Neurasthenia, toothache.

Yan(LO5) eye
Location: At the central point of the anterior surface of lobe.

Indications: Acute conjunctivitis, electric ophthalmia, hordeolum, pseudomyopia.

Neier(LO6) internal ear
Location: Middle portion on the posterior margin of lobe.

Indications: Internal auditory vertigo, tinnitus, poor hearing.

Mianjia(LO5,6i) cheek
Location: Between the points LO5 and LO6.

Indications: Facial paralysis, trigeminal neuralgia, acne, flat wart.

Biantaoti(LO7,8,9i) tonsil
Location: On the lower portion of the ear lobe, at the intersectio of the points LO7,8,9.

Indications: Tonsillitis, pharyngitis.

9. Points on the Posterior Surface of the Auricle

Erbeixin(P1) heart of posterior surface
Location: At the upper part of the back of lobe.

Indications: Palpitation, insomnia, dreaminess.

Erbeifei(P2) lung of posterior surface
Location: At the region from the posterior surface of point P3 to the root of ear.
Indications: Cough, asthma, skin itching.

Erbeipi(P3) spleen of posterior surface
Location: At the central point of the back of the ear.
Indications: Stomachache, indigestion, anorexia.

Erbeigan(P4) liver of posterior surface
Location: Lateral to P3.
Indications: Cholecystitis, cholelithiasis, hypochondriac pain.

Erbeishen(P5) kidney of posterior surface
Location: Lower portion of the back of ear.
Indications: Headache and dizziness, neurasthenia.

Erbeigou(PS) groove of posterior surface
Location: In a "Y" form depression of the back of ear, surrounded by antihelix, superior antihelix crus and inferior antihelix crus.
Indications: Hypertension, skin itching.

10. Points on the Ear Root

Shangergen(R1) upper ear root
Location: Upper part of the root of ear.
Indications: Epistaxis.

Ermigen(R2) root of ear vagus
Location: Corresponding to helix crus, at the root of ear and the juncture between ear back and mastoid process.
Indications: Cholecystitis, cholelithiasis, biliary ascariasis, nasal obstruction, tachycardia, abdominal pain, diarrhea.

Xiaergen(R3) ear root
Location: At the lower most rim of the root of ear.
Indications: Headache, hypotension, asthma, abdominal pain.

Chapter Four
Points of Scalp Acupuncture

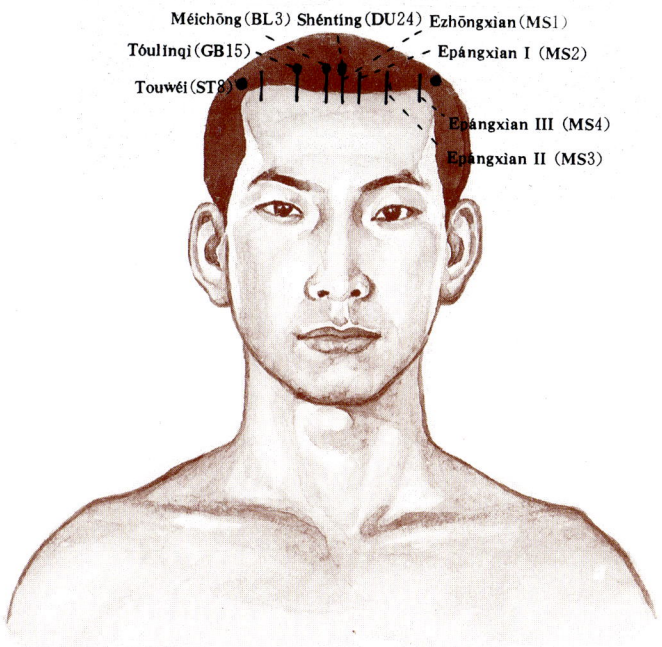
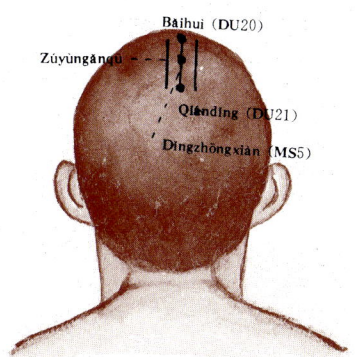
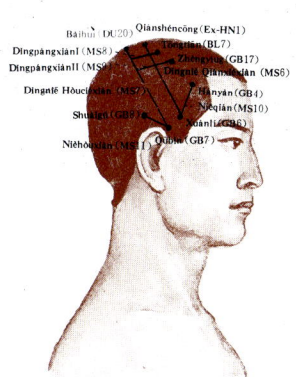

Fig. 24

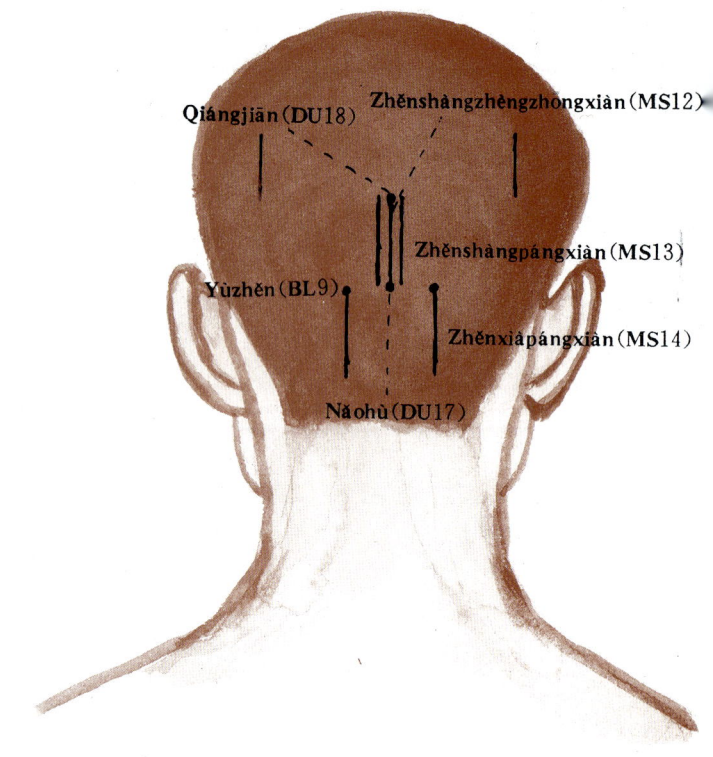

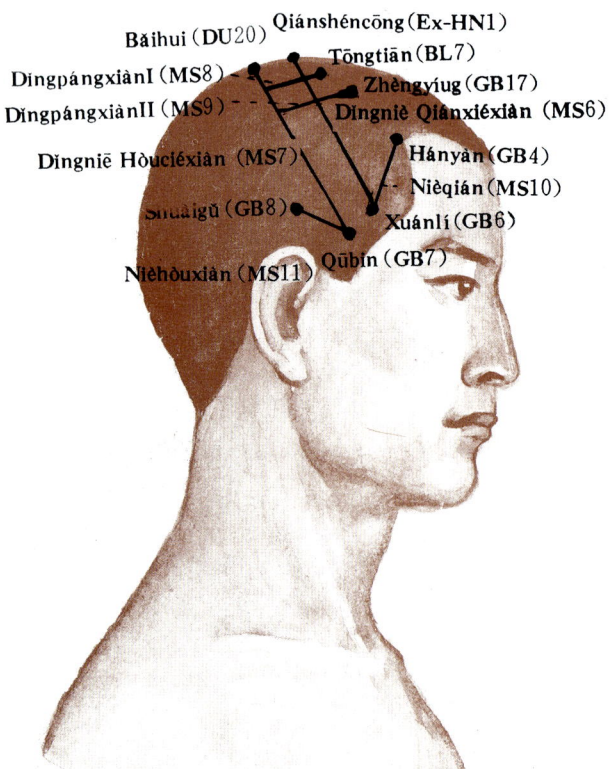

Fig. 25

The specific Areas on the Scalp

Ezhongxian(MS1) middle line of forehead
Location: At the middle of the frontal area, 1 cun from Shenting(DU24), straight down along the meridian.
Indications: Headache, dizziness, conjunctival congestion, epilepsy.
Method: Puncture subcutaneously downward and then twist the needle about 200 times per minute.

Epangxian(MS2) lateral line I of forehead
Location: Lateral to middle line of forehead, 1 cun from Meichong(BL3), straight down along the Meridian.
Indications: Allergic asthma, bronchitis, precordial pain, rheumatic heart disease, supraventricular paroxysmal tachycardia.
Method: Puncture subcutaneously 1 cun from Meichong with quick twisting method.

Epangxian II (MS3) lateral line II of forehead
Location: Lateral to latreal line I of forehead, 1 cun from Toulinqi(GB15), straight down along the meridian.
Indications: Pain due to acute or chronic gastritis, gastroduodenal ulcer, also effective for upper abdominal pain due to hepatopathy.

Epangxian III(MS4) lateral line III of forehead
Location: Lateal to lateral line II of forehead, 1 cun from the point, 0.75 cun medial to Touwei(ST8) straight down.
Indications: Dysfunctional uterine bleeding, also effective for frequency of micturition, emergency of urine, thirst and enuresis due to diabetes, impotency, emission, prolapse of uterine, lower abdominal pain, etc.

Dingzhongxian(MS5) middle line of vertex
Location: Along the middle of head from Baihui(DU20) to Qianding(DU21)
Indications: Headache, dizziness, aphasia due to apoplexy, coma, manic-depressive psychosis epilepsy.

Dingnieqianxiexian(MS6) anterior oblique line of vertex-temporal
Location: From Qianshencong(EX-HN1) obliquely to Xuanli(GB6)
Indications: The upper 1/5 mainly for lower limb paralysis; middle 2/5 for upper limb paralysis; and lower 2/5 for central facial paralysis, aphemia, salivation, cerebral arteriosclerosis.
Method: Puncture subcutaneously 1.5 cun from Qianshencong(EX-HN1) to Qubin(GB7) backwards.

Dingpangxian I (MS8) lateral line I of vertex
Location: 1.5 cun lateral to middle line of vertex, 1.6 cun from Tongtian(BL7), backward along the meridian.
Indications: Mainly sensory disturbance, upper 1/5 for lower bimb, middle 2/5 for upper limb, and lower 2/5 for head and face.

Dingpangxian II (MS9) lateral line II of vertex
Location: 2.25 cun lateral to middle line of vertex, 1.5 cun from Zhengying(GB17), backwards along the meridian.
Indications: Headache and vertigo.
Method: Puncture subcutaneously 1.5 cun from Zhengying(GB7) backwards.

Nieqianxian(MS10) anterior temporal line
Location: From Hanyan(GB4) to Xuanli(GB6).
Indications: Headache, pain in the outer canthus, tinnitus, epilepsy.
Method: Puncture from Hanyan(GB4) to Xuanli(GB6).

Niehouxian(MS11) posterior temporal line

Location: From Shuaigu(GB8) to Qubin(GB7).

Indications: Headache, vertigo, infantile convulsion etc..

Zhenshangzhenzhongxian(MS12) upper middle line of occiput

Location: At the middle of the occiput, one portion of Du meridians, from Qiangjian(DU18) to Naohu(DU12).

Indications: Headache, dizziness, stiffness of the neck and nape, manic-depressive psychosis, epilepsy.

Method: Puncture from Shuaigu(GB8) to Qubin(GB7).

Zhenshangpangxian(MS13) upper lateral line of occiput

Location: 0.5 cun lateral and parallel to upper middle line of occiput.

Indications: Cortical visual disturbance, cataract, myopia.

Method: Puncture subcutaneously 1.33 cun from the lower part upwards.

Zhenxiapangxian(MS14) lower lateral line of occiput

Location: Straight down from Yuzhen(BL9).

Indications: Cerebellar disorders, occipital headache, etc..

Method: Puncture subcutaneously 1.33 cun, from the upper part.

Chapter Five
Points of Hand Acupuncture

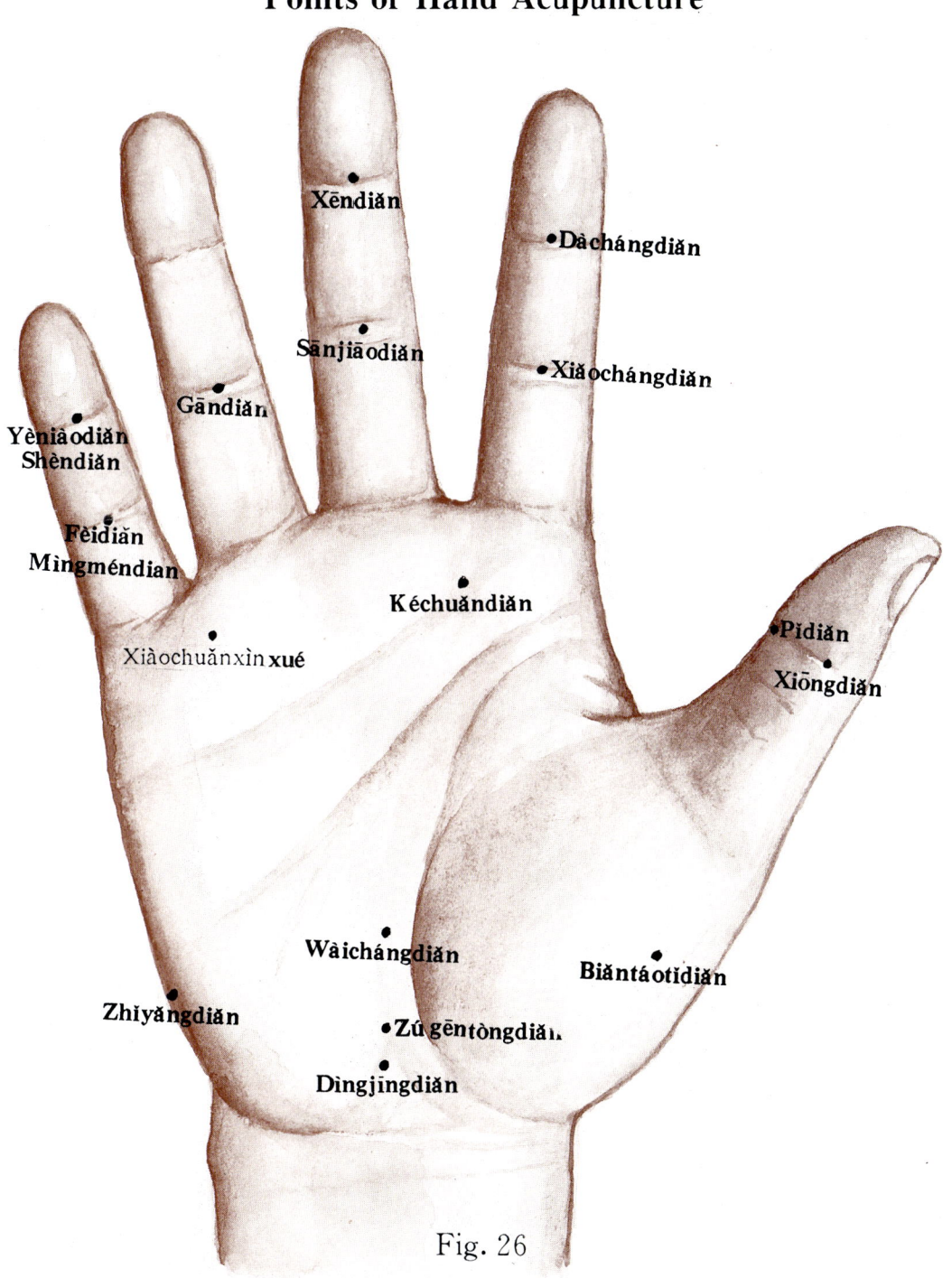

Fig. 26

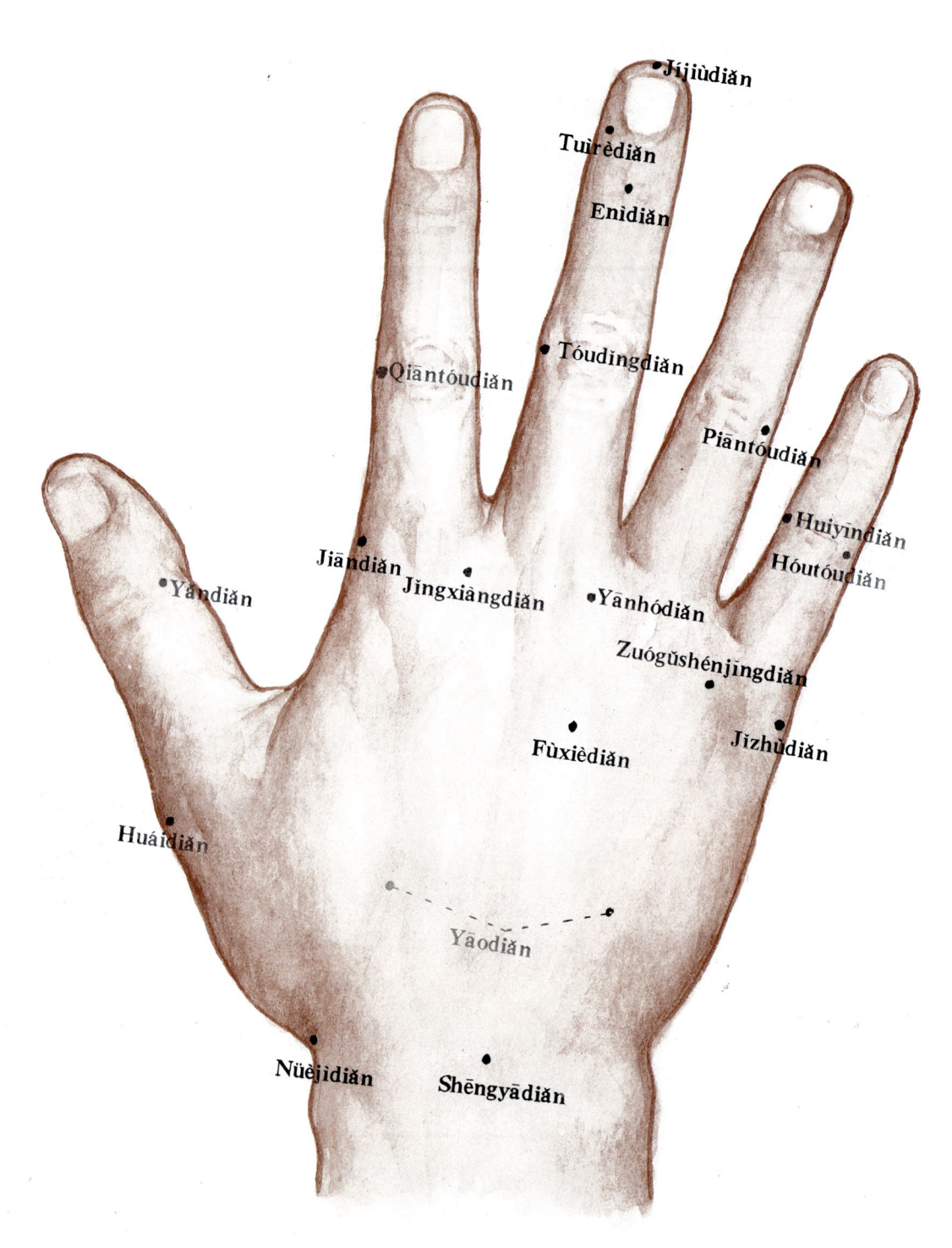

Fig. 27

Huaidian
Location: On the red-white border, radial side of the metacarpophalangeal joint of the thumb.
Indications: Sprain of ankle joint with pain.

Xiongdian
Location: On the red-white border, radial side of the pollical joint.
Indications: Chest pain, vomiting, diarrhea, epilepsy.

Yandian
Location: On the red-white border, ulnar side of the pollical joint.
Indications: Ophthalmic diseases, such as conjunctival congestion, ophthalmalgia, blurred vision, hordeolum, optic atrophy.

Jiandian
Location: On the red-white border, radial side of the metacarpophalangeal joint of the index finger.
Indications: Sprain of the shoulder joint, omalgia, scapulohumeral periarthritis.

Qiantoudian
Location: On the red-white border, radial side of the first metacarpophalangeal joint of the index finger.
Indications: Headache, gastric pain, vomiting, abdominal pain, diarrhea, appendicitis, omalgia, toothache.

Toudingdian
Location: On the red-white border, radial side of the first middle finger joint.
Indications: Parietal headache, dysmenorrhea.

Piantoudian
Location: On the red-white border, ulnar side of the first ring finger joint.
Indications: Migraine, intercostal neuralgia.

Huiyindian
Location: On the red-white border, radial side of the first little finger joint.
Indications: Dysmenorrhea, morbid vaginal discharge, pain in the perineum.

Houtoudian
Location: On the red-white border, ulnar side of the first little finger joint.
Indications: Headache in the occiput, sore-throat, tonsillitis, stiffness of the nape, pain in the shoulder and arm, pain in the cheek.

Jizhudian
Location: On the red-white border, ulnar side of the metacarpophalangeal joint of the little finger.
Indications: Lumbago, sprain of the lumbar joint, prolapse of lumbar intervertebral disc, coccyalgia and sacral pain, tinnitus, stuffy nose.

Zuogudian
Location: Between the fourth and fifth metacarpophalangealarticulations, near the former.
Indications: Lumbocrural pain, pain in the hip and buttock.

Yanhoudian
Location: Between the third and fourth metacarpophalangealarticulations, near the former.
Indications: Sore throat, tonsillitis, toothache, prosopalgia.

Jingxiangdian
Location: Between the second and third metacarpophalangealarticulations, near the former.

Indications: Stiff neck, swelling of the neck, sprain of theneck.

Yaotuidian

Location: On the dorsum of hand, 1.5 cun anterior to the crossstriation of the wrist, one is on the radial side of the secondextensor tendon, the other on the ulnar side of the fourthextensor tendon.

Indications: Lumbocrural pain.

Shengyadian

Location: At the midpoint of the the cross striation of thewrist.

Indications: Hypotension.

Enidian

Location: On the dorsum of hand, at the midpoint of the crossstriation of the second interphalangeal articulation of themiddle finger.

Indications: Hiccup.

Tuiredian

Location: On the dorsum of hand, and on the web of the radialside of the middle finger.

Indications: Fever, diarrhea.

Fuxiedian

Location: On the dorsum of hand, 1 cun anterior to the 3rd and4th metacarpophalangeal articulations.

Indications: Diarrhea.

Zhiyangdian

Location: 1 cun anterior to the ulnar of the cross striation ofthe wrist, and on the junction of the red and white skin.

Indications: Pruritus cutanea.

Weichangdian

Location: At the midpoint of the line connecting Laogong(PC8) andDaling(PC7).

Indications: Chronic gastritis, indigestion.

Xiaochuankesoudian

Location: On the ulnar side of the the metacarpophangealarticulation of the index.

Indications: Bronchitis, asthma, neurologic headache.

Yeniaodian

Location: On the palmar surface, at the midpoint of the crossstriation of the 2nd interphalangeal articulation of the littlefinger.

Indications: Enuresis, frequency of micturition.

Zugentongdian

Location: At the midpoint of Weichangdian and Daling(PC7).

Indications: Painful heels.

Niejidian

Location: On the junction of the first metacarpal bone and carpaljoint, radial side of the thenar.

Indications: Fever due to malaria.

Biantaotidian

Location: On the palmar surface, at the midpoint of the firstinterphalangeal articulation, on the ulnar side.

Indications: Tonsillitis, laryngitis.

Jijiudian

Location: On the tip of the middle finger, 0.2 cun near the nail.

Indications: Coma, heat apoplexy.

Dingjingdian
Location: On the palmar surface, on the junction of the thenar and hypothenar.

Indications: High fever, convulsion.

Pidian
Location: On the palmar surface, at the midpoint of the crossstriation of the interphalangeal articulation of the thumb.

Indications: Diarrhea, abdominal pain.

Xiaochangdian
Location: On the palmar surface, at the midpoint of the interphalangeal articulation between the first and second-phalanges of the index.

Indications: Diseases distributed to the small intestine.

Dachangdian
Location: On the palmar surface, at the midpoint of the interphalangeal articulation between the second and third-phalanges of the index.

Indications: Diarrhea, constipation.

Sanjiaodian
Location: On the palmar surface, at the midpoint of the interphalangeal articulation between the first and second-phalanges of the middle finger.

Indications: Disorders distributed to the chest, abdomen and pelvic cavity.

Xindian
Location: On the palmar surface, at the midpoint of the interphalangeal articulation between the second and third-phalanges of the middle finger.

Indications: Palpitation, precoridal pain.

Gandian
Location: On the palmar surface, at the midpoint of the interphalangeal articulation between the first and second-phalanges of the ring finger.

Indications: Pain in the hypochondriac region, epigastricdistention.

Feidian
Location: On the palmar surface, at the midpoint of the interphalangeal articulation between the first and second-phalanges of the little finger.

Indications: Cough, dyspnea, chest distress.

Mingmendian
Location: On the palmar surface, at the midpoint of the interphalangeal articulation between the second and third-phalanges of the little finger.

Indications: Lumbago, emission, impotency.

Shendian
Location and indications: The same as that of Miniaodian.

Xiaochuanxinxue
Location: On the palmar surface, on the junction between the 4th and 5th metacarpophalangeal articulations.

Indications: Asthma.

Chapter Six
Points of Eye Socket Acupuncture

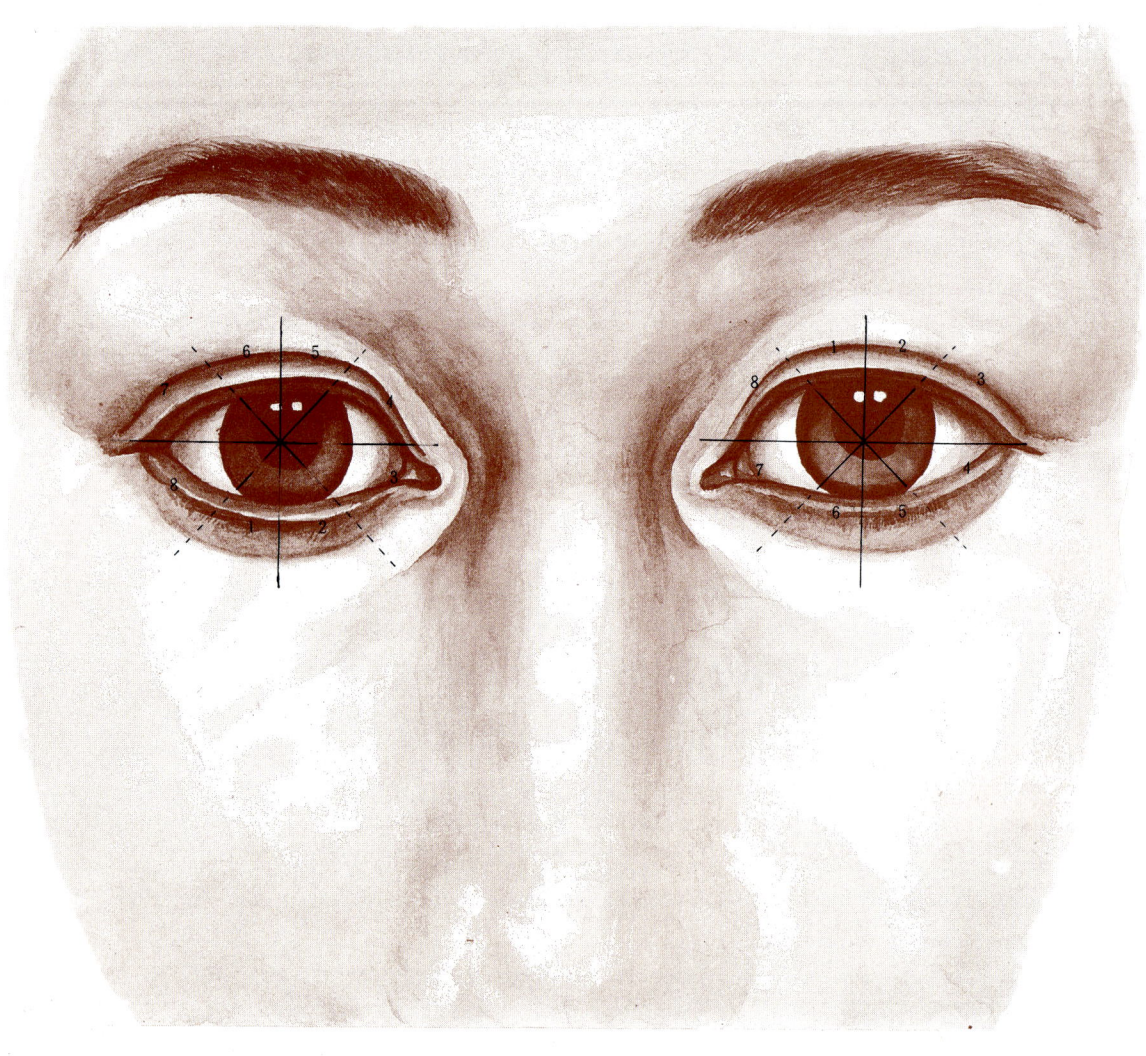

Fig. 28

The bulbus oculi is divided into 8 portions.

Method: Ask the patient to look straight ahead, make a horizontal line and a perpendicular line through the midpoint of pupil. Thus four quadrants are established. Every quadrant is divided into two parts equally. We then get 8 portions. The eye is described as a clock, then one portion owns 90 minutes.

The eight portions respectively attributive to the corresponding organs.

1. The first portion: lung and large intestine;
2. the second: kidney and bladder;
3. the third: the upper jiao;
4. the fourth: liver and gallbladder;
5. the fifth: the middle jiao;
6. the sixth: heart and small intestine;
7. the seventh: spleen and stomach;
8. the eighth: the lower jiao.

Chapter Seven
Points of Nasal Acupuncture

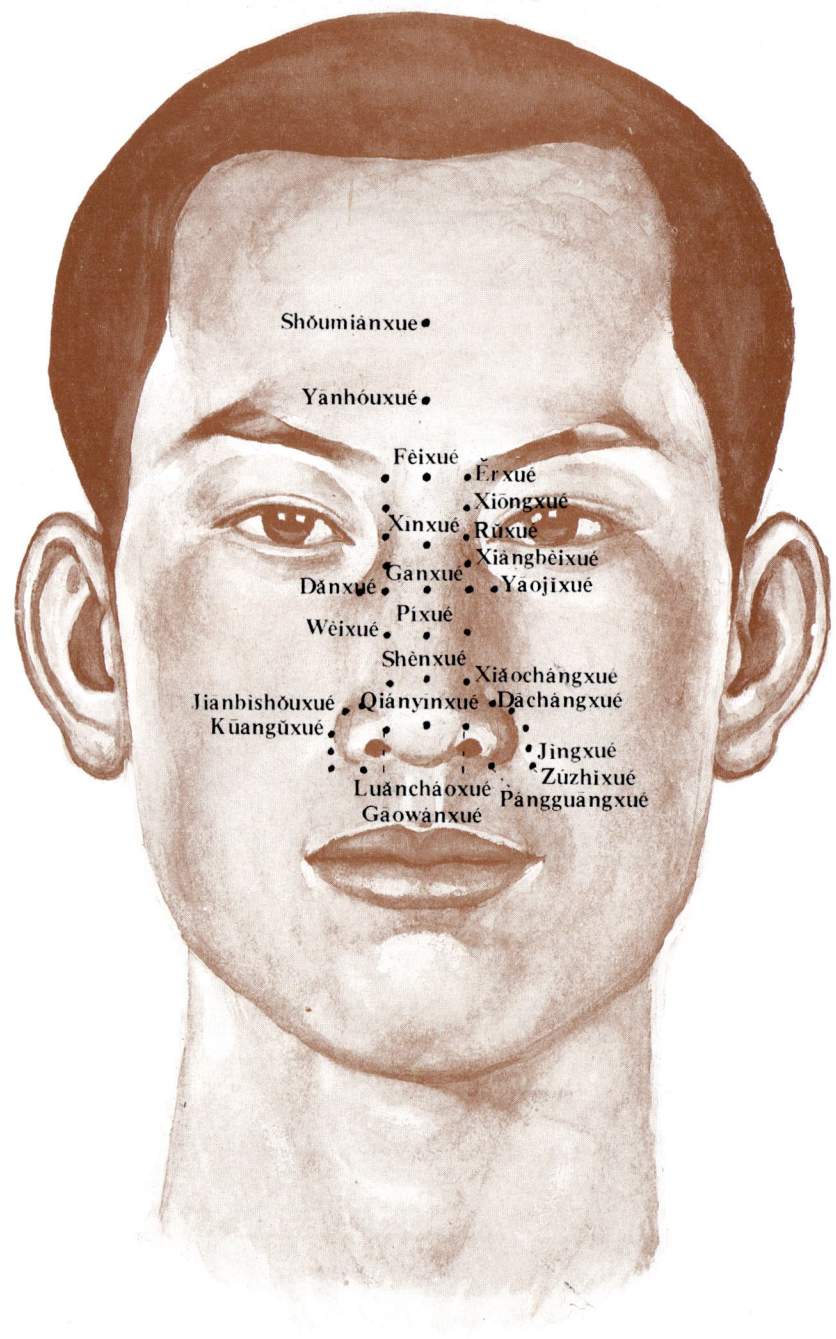

Fig. 29

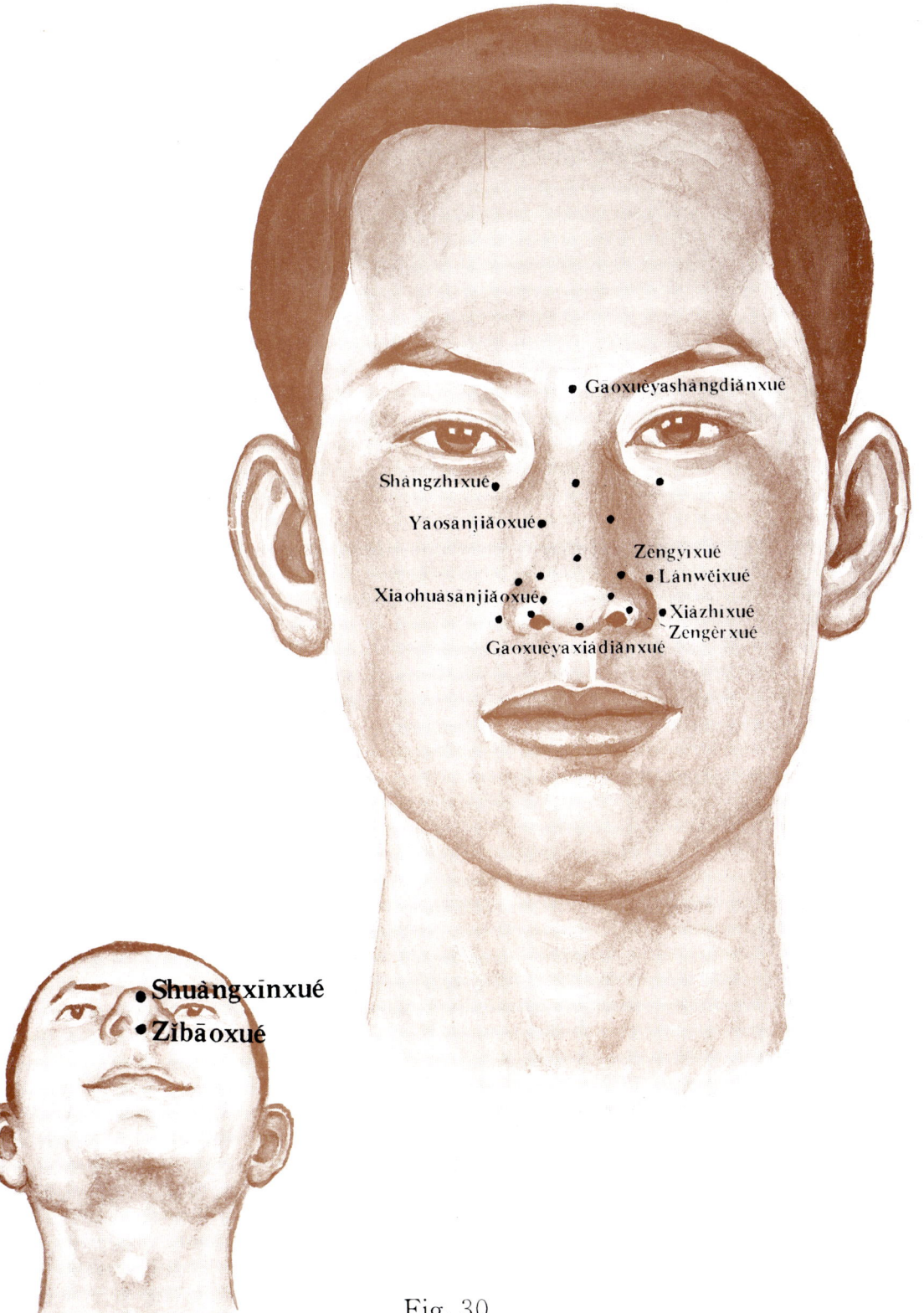

Fig. 30

There are three Point Lines in nasal point system. The first start from the central point of the forehead to the apex of nose, also known as anterior midline of nose.

Shoumianxue

Location: Central point of the forehead, midpoint of the line connecting ophryon and anterior hairline.

Yanhouxue

Location: Midpoint of the line connecting Shoumian and Fei

Feixue

Location: Just on the ophryon.

Xinxue

Location: Midpoint of the line connecting the inner canthi.

Ganxue

Location: Midpoint of the line connecting the points Xin and Pi.

Pixue

Location: On the anterior midline, midpoint of the line connecting the points Xin and Qianyin.

Shenxue

Location: On the anterior midline, midpoint of the line connecting the points Pi and Qianyin.

Qianyinxue, Shengzhiqi

Location: The apex of nose.

The second line starts from the height equal to the point Gan, to the lower extremity of ala nasi.

Danxue

Location: Just below the inner canthus, medial to Gan.

Weixue

Location: Below the point Dan, medial to Pi.

Xiaochangxue

Location: Below the point Wei, on the upper 1/3 of the ala nasi.

Dachangxue

Location: Below the point Xiaochang, at the central point of the ala nasi.

Pangguangxue

Location: Below the point Dachang, on the lower border of the ala nasi.

The third line starts from the medial extremity of eyebrow, goes down 0.1-0.2 cun lateral to the second line, and then to the lower border of nose.

Erxue

Location: Medial extremity of the eyebrow.

Xiongxue

Location: Below the superciliary arch, superior and medial to the orbit

Ruxue

Location: Superior to Jingming(BL1).

Xiangbeixue

Location: Below Jingming(BL1).

Yaojixue

Location: Medial to zygomatic bone, lateral to point Gan.

Jianbishouxue
Location: Below Yaoji, lateral to the upper part of the ala nasi.

Jingxue
Location: Below the point Kuangu.

Zuzhixue
Location: Below the point Jing, lateral to Pangguang.

Kuangu
Location: Below the point Jianbishou.

Some new-found points

Gaoxueyashangdianxue
Location: The same as Yintang(EX-HN3)

Yaosanjiaoxue
Location: On the lower portion of nasal bone, the maximum is just below the point Xin.

Xiaohuasanjiaoxue
Location: The maximum is just below that of Yaosanjiao.

Gaoxueyaxiadianxue
Location: Slightly below the apex of nose.

Shangzhixue
Location: Below the point Jianbishou.

Lanweixue
Location: On the lateral superior portion of ala nasi.

Xiazhixue
Location: The same as the point Jing.

Chuangxinxue
Location: On the anterior midline, medial to the upper border of the nostril.

Zengyixue
Location: The fossa on the medial border of the ala nasi.

Zengerxue
Location: On the upper border of the nostril, just below the point Zengyi.

Zibaoxue
Location: Slightly below the nasal septum, superior to Shuigou(DU26).

Chapter Eight
Points of Mouth Acupuncture

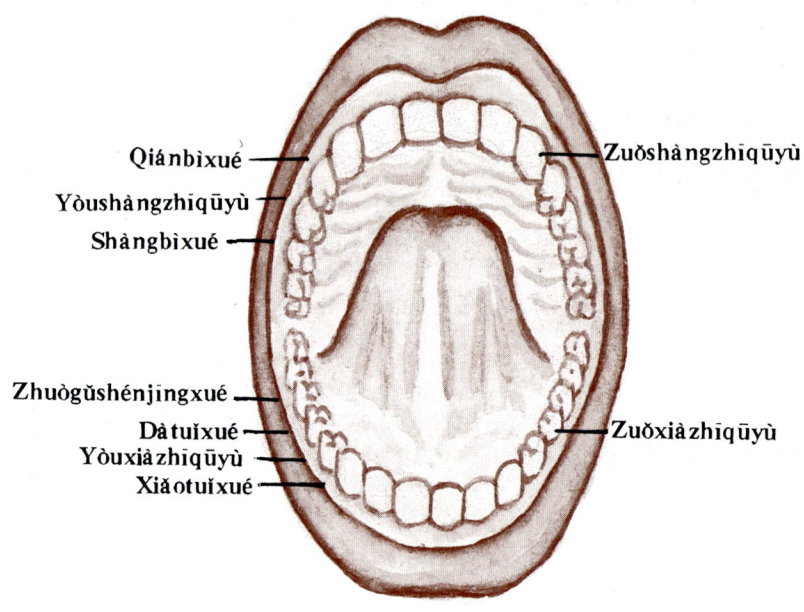

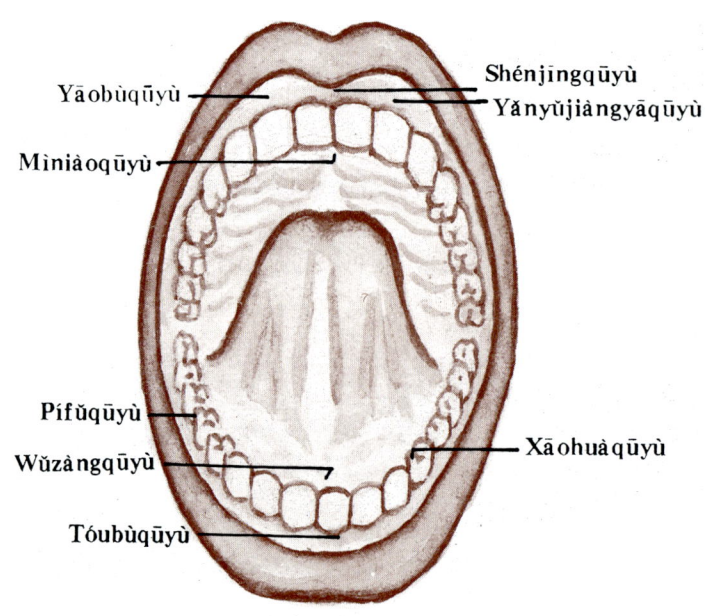

Fig. 31

Shangzhiquyu, upper limb region

Location: On the tunica mucosa oris between the lateral inciesr and the first molar tooth of the left maxillary.

Indications: Pain and sprain of the joints of the upper limb, hemiparalysis from cerebrovascular accident.

1) Shangbixue, upper arm

Location: On the tunica mucosa oris between the first and the second molar teeth, left to the maxilla.

Indications: Pain in the shoulder and upper arm.

2) Qianbixue, forearm

Location: On the tunica mucosa oris between the left canine tooth and the first bicuspid premolar of the left maxilla.

Indications: Swelling pain in the forearm.

Xiazhiqu, lower limb region

Location: On the tunica mucosa oris among the mandibular canine teeth and the third molar tooth.

Indications: Sprain of lower limb joints, pain, sciatica, sequel of infantile paralysis, equel from cerebrovascular accident.

1) Zuogushenjing, sciatic nerve

Location: Between the first and the second molar teeth of the left mandible. On the tunica mucosa oris below the gingivae.

Indications: Sciatica.

2) Datui, thigh

Location: Between the second bicuspid premolar and the first molar tooth of the left mandible. On the tunica mucosa oris below the gingivae.

Indications: Cold pain or distention in the thigh.

3) Xiaotuixue, lower leg

Location: Between the canine teeth and the first bicuspid premolar of the left mandible. On the tunica mucosa oris below the gingivae.

Indications: Systremma.

Shenjingquyu, nerve region

Location: On the tunica mucosa oris above the gingivae of central incisors of the maxillary.

Indications: Prosopalgia, facial paralysis.

Toubuquyu, head region

Location: On the tunica mucosa oris below the gingivae of central incisors of the maxillary.

Indications: nervous headache, stiffneck.

Miniaoquyu, urination region

Location: On the membrana propria above the gingivae of central incisors of the maxillary.

Indications: Frequency of micturition, urodynia, emission, enuresis, dysmenorrhea.

Xiaohuaquyu, digestion region

Location: On the membrana propria below the gingivae of the canine teeth of the left mandible.

Indications: Acute gastroenteritis, indigestion, diarrhea, abdominal pain, gastric pain.

Wuzangquyu, viscera region

Location: On the membrana propria below the gingivae of the lateral incisor of the right mandible.
Indications: Cough, dyspnea, palpitation.

Yanjijiangyaquyu, eye & step-down region

Location: On the tunica mucosa oris above the gingivae of the lateral incisor of left maxillary.
Indications: Ophthalmic disorders, hypertension.

Yaobuquyu, lumbar region

Location: On the tunica mucosa oris above the gingivae of the lateral incisor of right maxillary.
Indications: Sprain of the lumbar joint; lumbar muscle strain.

Pifuquyu, skin region

Location: On the tunica mucosa oris above the gingivae of the first molar tooth of the left mandible.
Indications: Pruritus cutanea, paralysis.

Chapter Nine
Points of Tongue Acupuncture

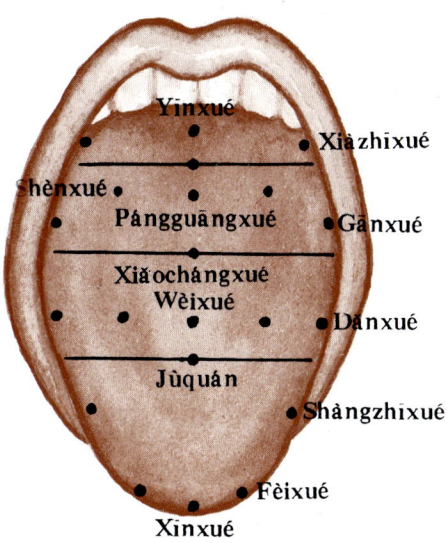

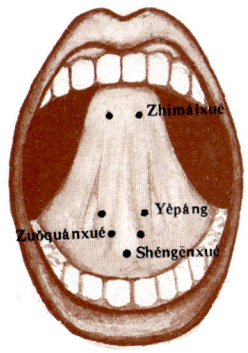

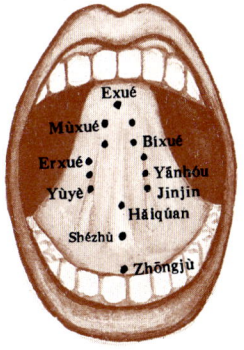

Fig. 32

Xinxue
Location: On the tongue tip.
Indications: Diseases belonging to Heart Meridian.

Feixue
Location: On the lingual surface, 0.3 cun lateral to Xinxue.
Indications: Diseases belonging to Lung Meridian.

Weixue
Location: At the central point of the lingual surface, 1 cun posterior to Xinxue.
Indications: Diseases belonging to Stomach Meridian.

Pixue
Location: On the lingual surface, 0.4 cun lateral to Weixue.
Indications: Diseases belonging to Spleen Meridian.

Danxue
Location: On the lingual surface, 0.8 cun lateral to Weixue.
Indications: Diseases belonging to Gallbladder Meridian.

Ganxue
Location: On the lingual surface, 0.5 cun lateral to Weixue.
Indications: Diseases belonging to Liver Meridian.

Xiaochangxue
Location: On the lingual surface, 0.3 cun posterior to Weixue.
Indications: Diseases belonging to Small Intestine Meridian.

Pangguangxue
Location: On the lingual surface, 0.3 cun posterior to Xiaochangxue.
Indications: Diseases belonging to Bladder Meridian.

Shenxue
Location: On the lingual surface, 0.4 cun lateral to Pangguangxue.
Indications: Diseases belonging to Kidney Meridian.

Dachangxue
Location: On the lingual surface, 0.2 cun posterior to Pangguangxue.
Indications: Diseases belonging to Large Intestine Meridian.

Yinxue
Location: On the root of the tongue, 0.2 cun posterior to Dachangxue.
Indications: Diseases relating to the external urethral orifice and the anus.

Juquan
Location: At the central point of lingual surface, 2 cun anterior to Weixue.
Indications: Diabetes, stiff tongue.

Shangzhixue
Location: On the lingual margin, between Feixue and Danxue.
Indications: Upper limb diseases.

Xiazhixue

Location: On the root of tongue, near the lingual margin, 1 cun lateral to Yinxue.

Indication: Paralysis.

Sanjiaoxue

Location: Make three transverse lines respectively through Juquan, Xiaochangxue and Dachangxue. The portion between the tongue tip and Juquan named Shangjiao; the portion between Juquan and Xiaochangxue named Zhongjiao; Xiajiao locates between Xiaochangxue and Dachangxue.

Indications: Diseases attributive to Sanjiao Meridian.

Exue

Location: On the dorsum linguae, 0.3 cun below the tongue tip when the tongue twirls upwards.

Indications: Headache and dizziness.

Muxue

Location: On the dorsum linguae, 0.3 cun obliquely below Exue.

Indications: Conjunctival congestion with ophthalmalgia.

Bixue

Location: On the dorsum linguae, in the region between the lingual margin and the sublingual vein, 0.3 cun below Muxue.

Indications: Stuffy nose, rhinorrhea with turbid discharge.

Erxue

Location: On the dorsum linguae, 0.2 cun obliquely below Bixue.

Indications: Tinnitus, deafness.

Yanhouxue

Location: On the dorsum linguae, 0.2 cun below Erxue.

Indication: Sore-throat.

Haiquan

Location: Just on the frenulum linguae.

Indications: Hiccup, diabetes.

JinjinYuye

Location: Two veins lateral to the frenulum linguae, the left named Jinjin, the right, Yuye.

Indications: Stomatocace, glossitis, tonsillitis, vomiting, dysmenorrhea.

Shenzhu

Location: On the midpoint, the lower part of the dorsum linguae.

Indications: Double tongue, swelling tongue.

Zhongju

Location: On the conjunction of the tongue root and the palate.

Indications: Dry tongue, aphasia due to apoplexy.

New Found Points

Shengen

Location: On the fossa of the root of frenulum linguae.

Indications: Hypertension, cerebral thrombosis.

Zuoquan

Location: On the carunclae lateral to the frenulum linguae, near the orifice of the sublingual ducts.
Indications: Sequel from apoplexy.

Yepang

Location: On the dorsum linguae, 0.3 cun lateral to the sublingual vein.
Indications: Hypertension, sequel from cerebrovascular accident.

Zhimai

Location: On the root of the tongue, lateral to the sublingual vein.
Indications: Hypertension, equel from cerebrovascular accident.

Chapter Ten
Points of Chest Massage Acupuncture

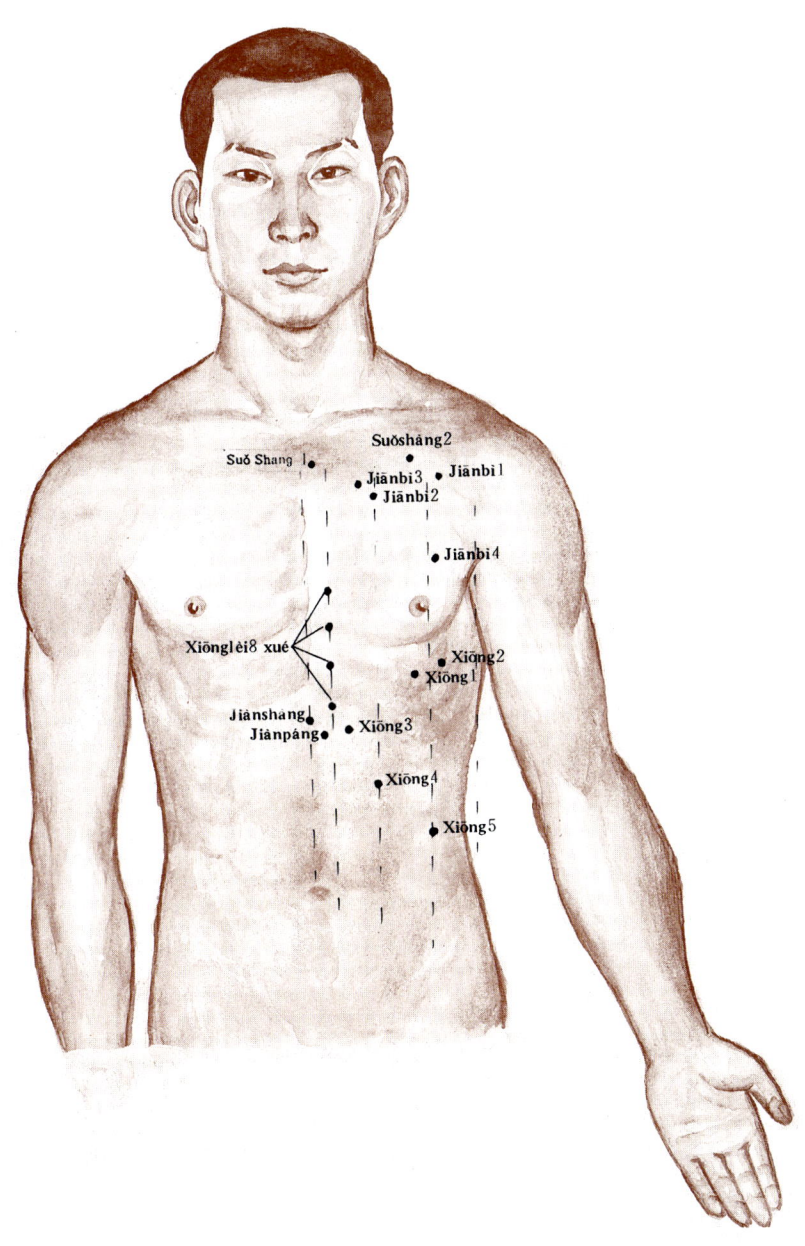

Fig. 33

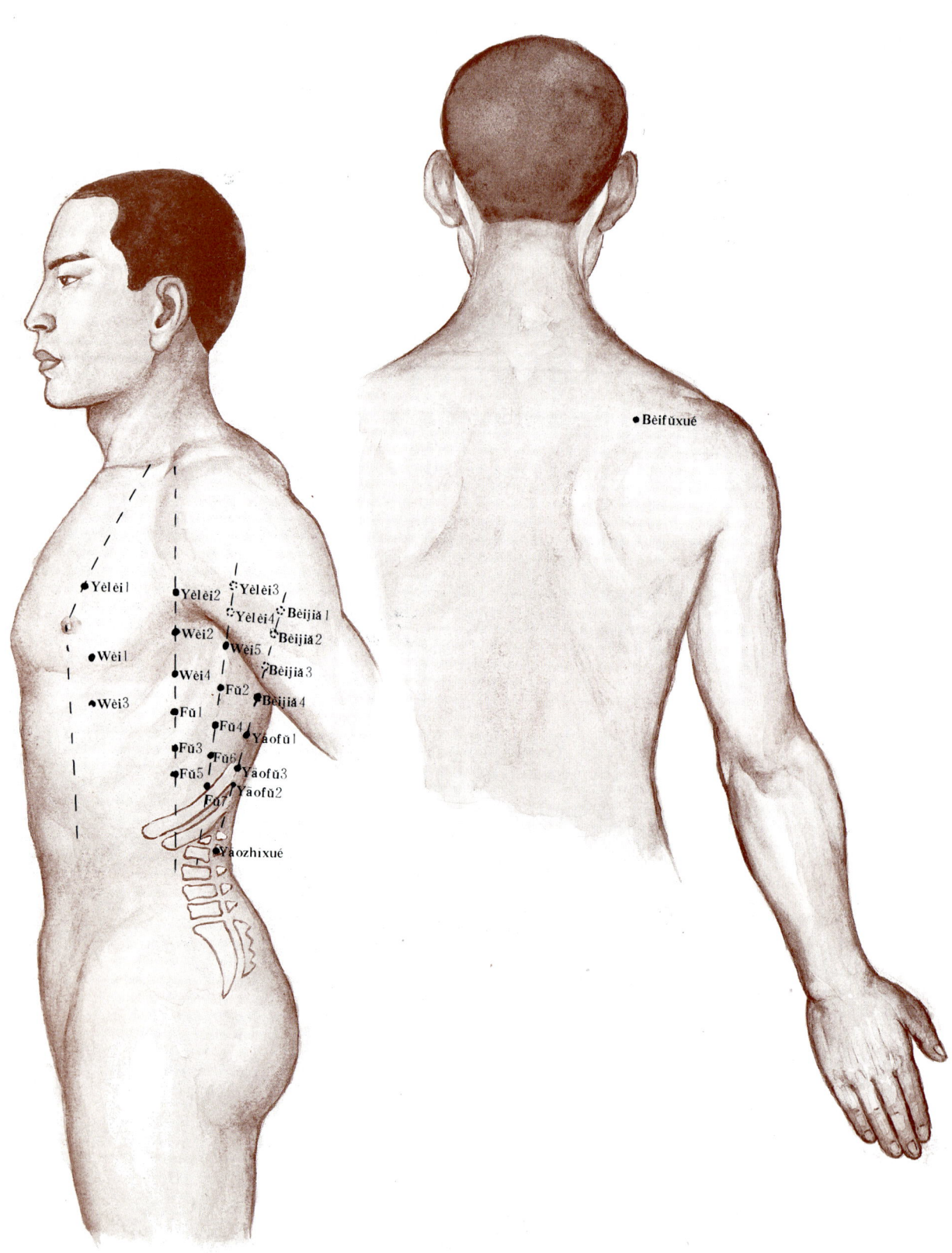

Fig. 34

1. Points on the lateral portion of the chest wall

Wei1

Location: On the lower margin of the 5th rib, 1 finger lateral to the midclavicular line.

Wei2

Location: At the intersectio of the anterior axillary line and the lower margin of the 5th rib.

Wei3

Location: On the lower margin of the 6th rib, 1 finger lateral to the midclavicular line.

Wei4

Location: At the intersectio of the anterior axillary line and the lower margin of the 6th rib.

Wei5

Location: At the intersectio of the middle axillary line and the lower margin of the 6th rib.

The above five points are applied for stomachache, gastric pain, palpitation, vomiting, nausea, etc.

Fu1

Location: At the intersectio of the anterior axillary line and the lower margin of the 7th rib.

Fu2

Location: At the intersectio of the middle axillary line and the lower margin of the 7th rib.

Fu3

Location: At the intersectio of the anterior axillary line and the lower margin of the 8th rib.

Fu4

Location: At the intersectio of the middle axillary line and the lower margin of the 8th rib.

Fu5

Location: At the intersectio of the anterior axillary line and the lower margin of the 9th rib.

Fu6

Location: At the intersectio of the middle axillary line and the lower margin of the 9th rib.

Fu7

Location: At the intersectio of the middle axillary line and the lower margin of the 10th rib.

The above seen point are applied for abdominal pain, hepatic disorders, and dysmenorrhea, etc.

Yelei1

Location: At the intersectio of midclavicular line and the lower margin of the 3rd rib.

Yelei2

Location: At the intersectio of the anterior axillary line and the lower margin of the fourth rib.

Yelei3

Location: At the intersectio of middle axillary line and the lower margin of the 4th rib.

Yelei4

Location: At the intersectio of middle axillary line and the lower margin of the 5th rib.

The above four points are applied for pain in the axillary region.

Beijia1
Location: At the intersectio of posterior axillary line and the lower margin of the 5th rib.
Beijia2
Location: At the intersectio of posterior axillary line and the lower margin of the 6th rib.
Beijia3
Location: At the intersectio of posterior axillary line and the lower margin of the 7th rib.
Beijia4
Location: At the intersectio of posterior axillary line and the lower margin of the 8th rib.

The above four points are applied for scapulalgia and backache, and soft-tissue injury.

Yaofu1
Location: At the intersectio of posterior axillary line and the lower margin of the 9th rib.
Yaofu2
Location: At the intersectio of posterior axillary line and the lower margin of the 10th rib.
Yaofu3
Location: At the intersectio of posterior axillary line and the lower margin of the 11th rib.
Yaofu4
Location: At the intersectio of scapular line and the lower margin of the 11th rib.

The above four points are used for lumbosacral pain, lumbar injury, distention of the abdomen, dysmenorrhea, etc.

Beifuxue
Location: On the spine of scapula, two fingers' breadth below the central point.
Indications: Colic due to ascariasis of biliary tract, abdominal pain, omalgia and backache, pain in the elbow and forearm, stiffneck.

Yaozhixue
Location: At the intersectio of the lateral margin of sacrospinal muscle and the transverse line through the epiphysis of the 12th rib.
Indications: Sprain of lumbosacral region, pain and numbness in the lower extremities, abdominal pain.

(2) Points on the anterior portion of the chest wall

Suoshang1
Location: On the sternoclavicular articulation, superior border of the medial extremity of the clavicle.
Indications: Palpitation, migraine, otopathy.

Suoshang2
Location: 1 finger medial to the midpoint of the superior border of the clavicle.

Indications: Migraine, palpitation, spasm of the diaphragm, scapulalgia, pain in the upper limb, stiffneck.

Jianbi1
Location: Below the clavicle, one finger lateral to midclavicular line.

Indications: Numbness and pain in the arm, omalgia, tremor, stiffneck.

Jianbi2
Location: Below the clavicle, one finger medial to midclavicular line.

Indications: Omalgia and pain in the ulnar border of the posterior area of the arm.

Jianbi3
Location: Between the clavicle and the 1st rib, on the parasternal line.

Indications: Omalgia and pain in the radial border of the posterior area of the arm.

Jianbi4
Location: On the lower border of the 2nd rib, slightly lateral to midclavicular line.

Indications: Omalgia and pain in the posterior area of the arm.

Xiong1
Location: On the lower border of the 4th rib, 1 finger medial to midclavicular line.

Indications: Pain in the chest and hypochondriac region, intercostal neuralgia, palpitation.

Xiong2
Location: On the lower border of the 4th rib, 1 finger lateral to midclavicular line.

Indications: Chest pain in the lower region, intercostal neuralgia.

Xiong3
Location: The intersectio of the costal arch and parasternal line.

Indications: Pain in the lower chest and costal arch.

Xiong4
Location: The intersectio of the costal arch and midclavicular line.

Indications: Pain in the liver and hypochondriac region.

Xionglei
Location: On the inferior horns of the sternocostal joints, there are 8 such points on both sides from the 2nd to the 5th ribs.

Jianshang
Location: Just on the xiphisternal synchondrosis.

Indications: Dizziness, headache especially in the forehead.

Jianpang
Location: On the junction of the costal arch and xiphoid process.

Indication: Epigastric pain, vomiting.

Chapter Eleven
Points of Facial Acupuncture

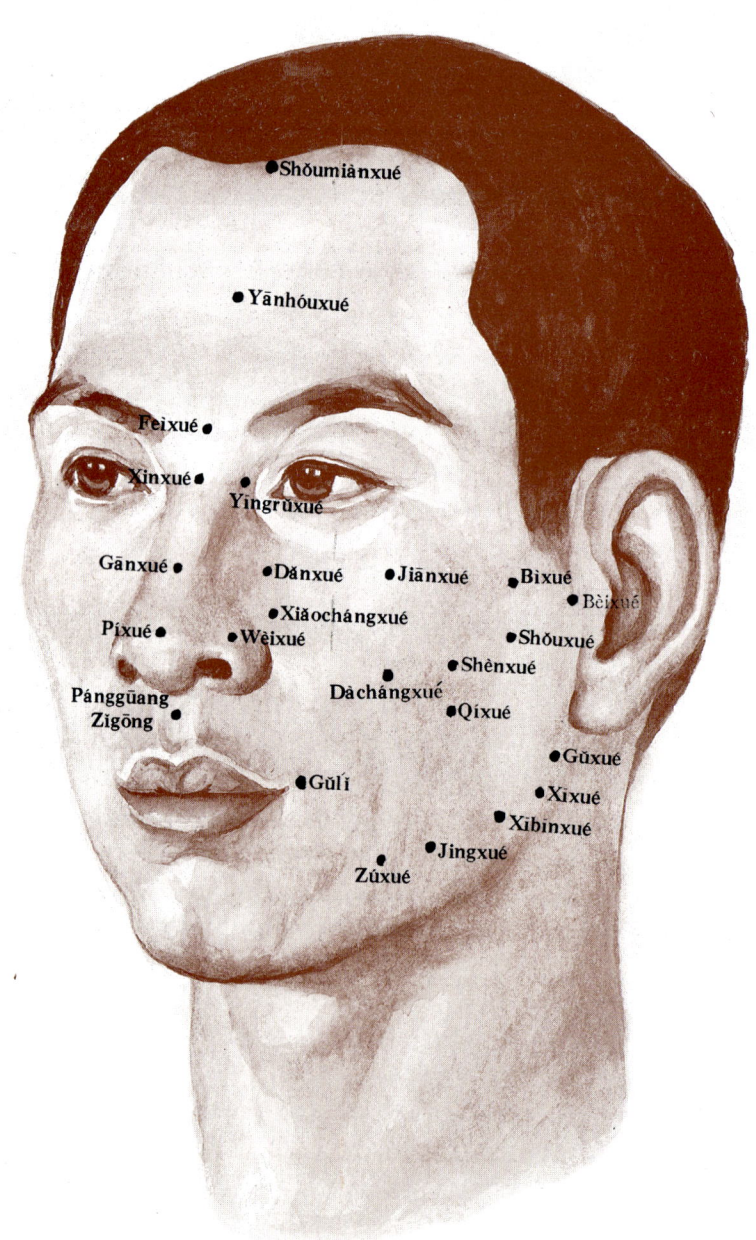

Fig. 35

Shoumianxue

Location: At the central point of the forehead.

Indications: Headache, dizziness.

Féixue, Yintang(EX-HN3)

Location: At the midpoint of the line connecting the medial extremity of the eyebrows.

Indication: Cough.

Yanhouxue

Location: Midpoint of the line connecting Shoumian and Fei.

Indication: Sore-throat.

Xinxue

Location: Midpoint of the line connecting the inner canthi.

Indication: Palpitation.

Ganxue

Location: Below the point Xin, on the lower border of the nasal bone, which connects with nasal cartilages.

Indications: Irritability, jaundice, hypochondriac pain.

Pixue, Suliao(DU24)

Location: On the apex of nose.

Indications: Anorexia, indigestion.

Pangguangxue

Location: At the midpoint of nasolabial groove.

Indications: Dysmenorrhea.

Danxue

Location: Lateral to the point Gan, just below the inner canthus, on the lower border of the dorsum of nose.

Indications: Nausea, vomiting.

Weixue

Location: Lateral to the point Pi, at the central point of ala nasi.

Indications: Gastric pain.

Yingru

Location: At the midpoint of the line connecting the point Xin and the inner canthus.

Indications: Hypogalactia.

Xiaochang

Location: Lateral to the midpoint of the line connecting the points Dan and Wei.

Indications: Diarrhea.

Dachangxue

Location: Just below the outer canthus, on the lower border of zygomatic bone.

Indications: Constipation, abdominal pain, diarrhea.

Shenxue

Location: Intersectio of the horizontal line through ala nasi and the perpendicular line through Taiyang(EX-HN5).

Indications: Oliguria, urodynia.

Qixue

Location: 0.3 cun below the point Shen.

Indications: Abdominal pain.

Beixue, Tinggong(SI19)

Location: 1.0 cun lateral and posterior to the central point of cheek.

Indication: Lumbago.

Jianxue

Location: Just below the outer canthus, lateral to the point Dan.

Indication: Omalgia with limitation of activity.

Shoumian

Location: Just below the point Bi, on the lower border of zygomatic arch.

Indications: Swelling pain in the hand.

Bimian

Location: Lateral to the point Jian, posterior to Xiaguan(ST7).

Indications: Swelling pain in the shoulder and arm.

Guxue 1

Location: Near Dicang(ST4), 0.5 cun lateral to the angulus oris.

Indications: Pain in the medial portion of the thigh.

Guxue 2

Location: On the junction of the upper 1/3 and middle 1/3 of the line connecting ear lobe and angulus mandibula.

Indications: Sprain of the thigh.

Xixue

Location: On the junction of the lower 1/3 and middle 1/3 of the line connecting the ear lobe and angulus mandibula.

Indication: Gonalgia.

Xibinxue, Jiache(ST6)

Location: On the cheek, one finger breadth (middle finger) anterior to mandibular angle., in the depression where the masseter muscle is prominent.

Indications: Injury of the knee joint.

Jingxue

Location: Anterior to the angulus mandibula, superior border of the mandible.

Indications: Sprain of ankle joint, systremma.

Zuxue

Location: Anterior to the point Jing, just below the outer canthus, on the superior border of the mandible.

Indication: Swelling pain in the foot.

Chapter Twelave
Points of Lateral Aspect Second Metacarpal Bone Acupuncture

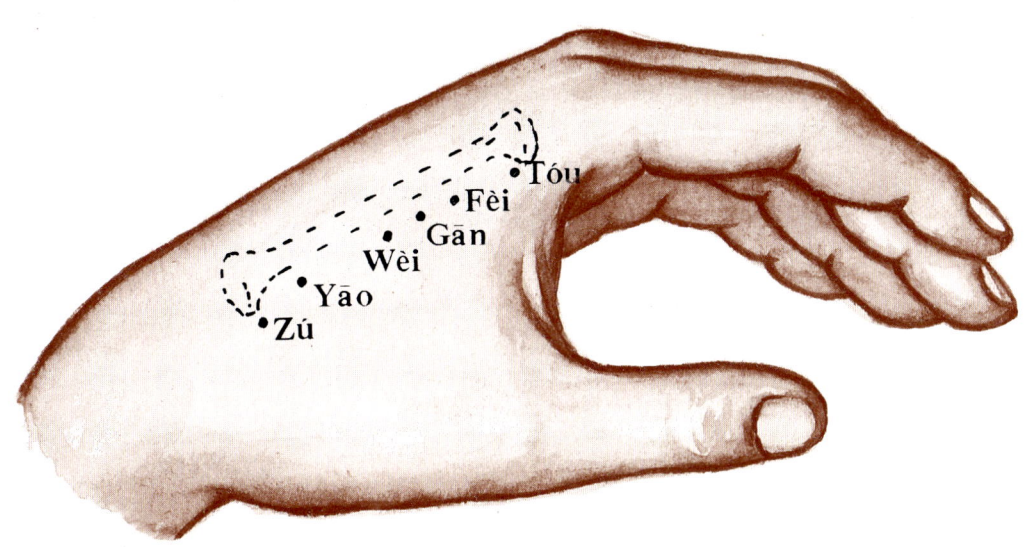

Fig. 36

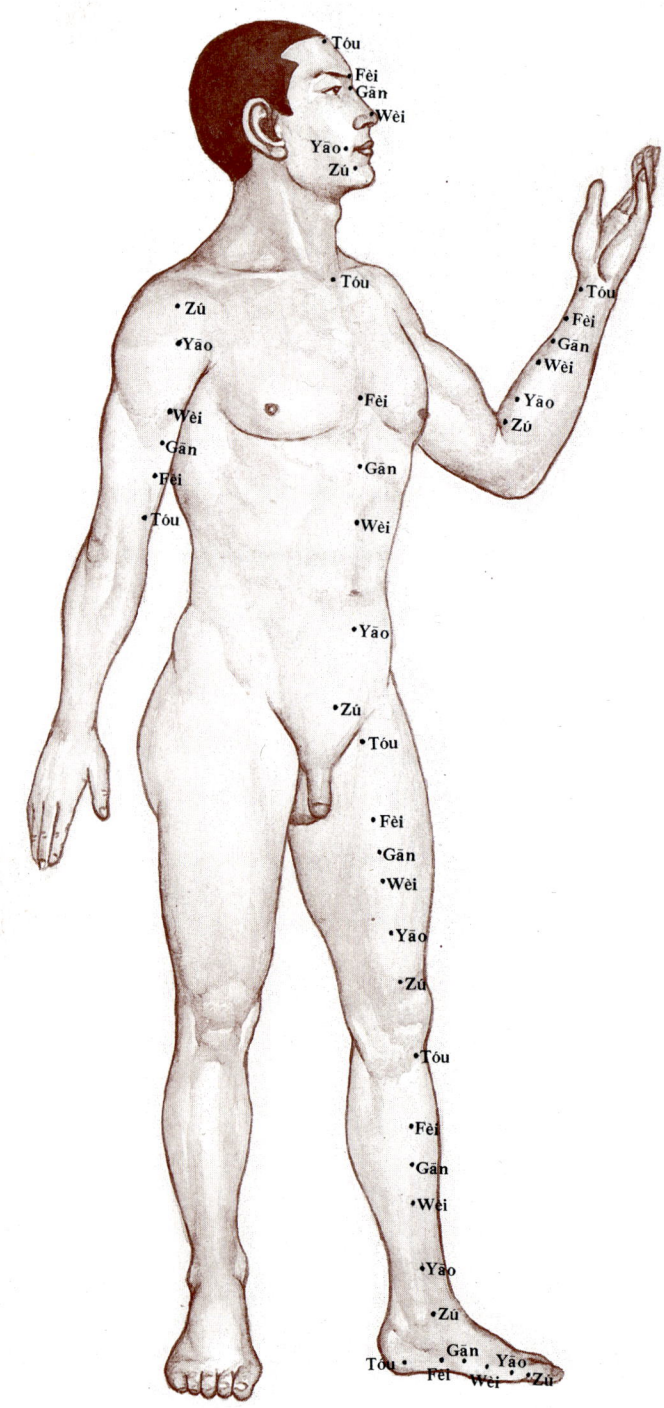

Fig. 37

Tou

Location: At the intersectio between the radial border of crossstriation of the palm and the second metacarpal bone.

Zu

Location: At the junction of the first and second metacarpalbones.

Wei

Location: At the midpoint of the line connecting the points Tou and Zu.

Fei

Location: At the midpoint of the line connecting the points Tou and Wei.

Gan

Location: At the midpoint of the line connecting the points Wei and Fei.

Yao

Location: At the intersectio of the anterior 1/3 and middle 1/3 of the line connecting Zu and Wei.

Qizhou

Location: At the intersectio of the middle 1/3 and posterior 1/3 of the line connecting Zu and Wei.

Chapter Thirteen
Points of Foot Acupuncture

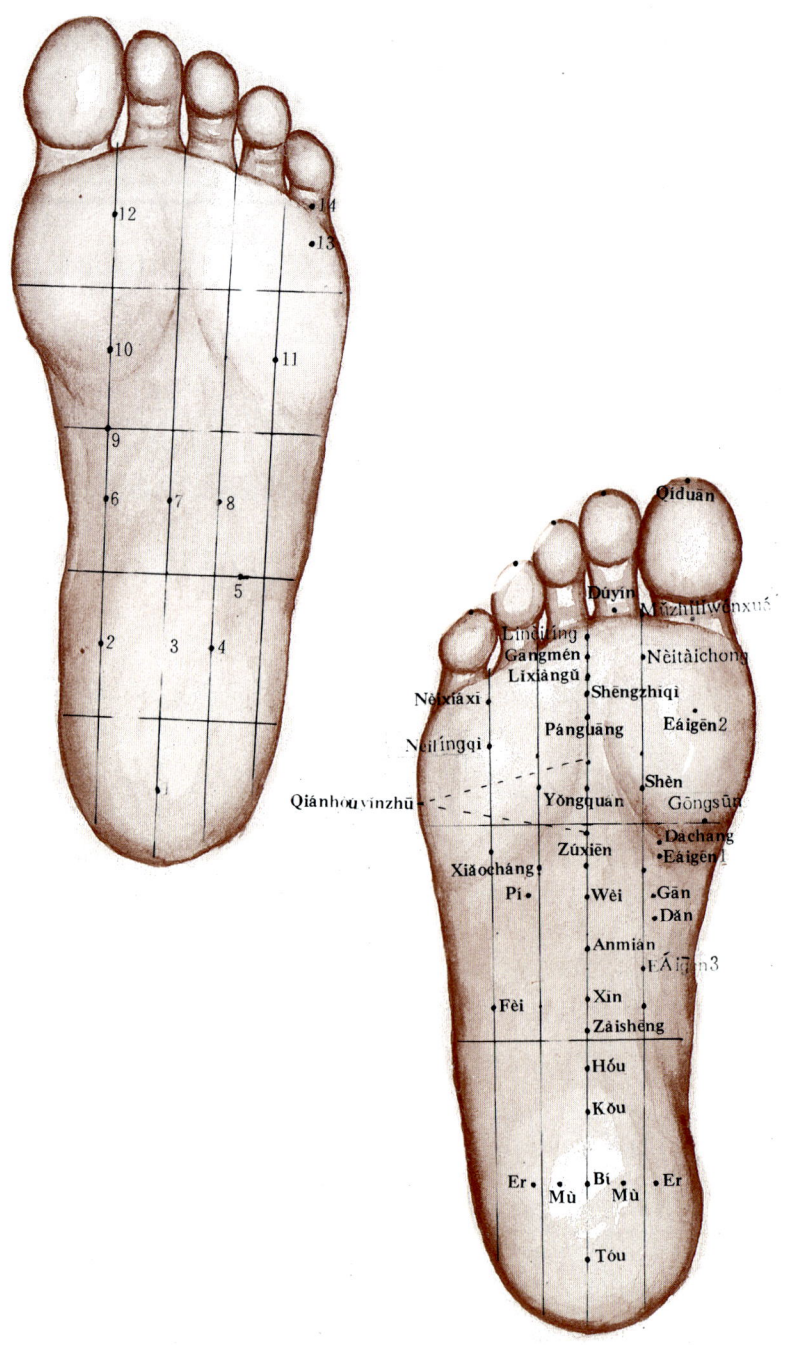

Fig. 38

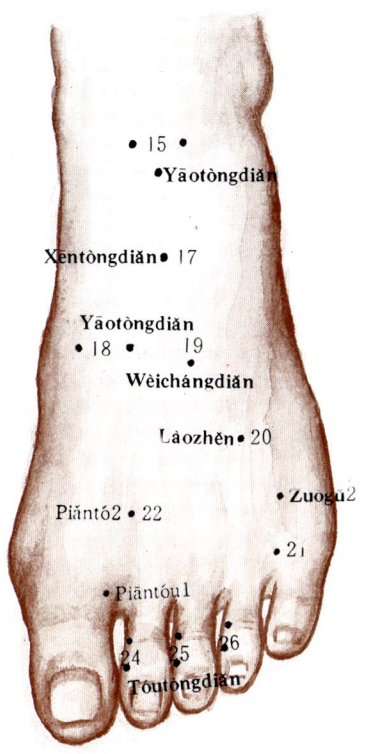

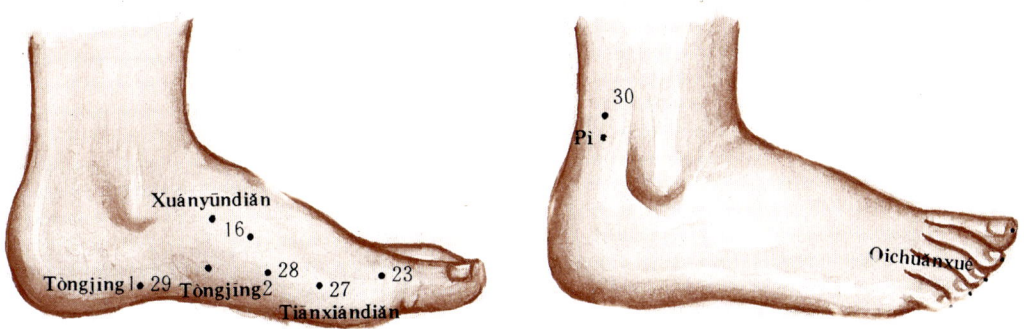

Fig. 39

Special bone proportional measurement:

On the plantar surface, the length between the midpoint of the posterior border of the heel and the web connecting the 2nd and 3rd toes, which is also named the mid-line, is divided into 10 portions, each portion as one cun; the length between the tip of the external malleolus and the lateral border of the planta (which is a perpendicular line) is taken as 3 cun; the length between the tip of the medial malleolus and the medial border of the planta (which is a perpendicular line) is taken as 3 cun; the widest length of the heel is taken as 3 cun; the length between the lines connecting the webs among the neighboring toes and posterior border of the heel (parallel to the mid-line) taken respectively as 1 cun.

Points on the planta

Touxue

Location: On the mid-line of the planta, 1 cun anterior to the midpoint of the junction of the red and white skin of the heel. Indications: Headache, toothache. Muxue

Location: 0.6 cun lateral to the point Bixue.

Indications: Acute and chronic ophthalmic diseases.

Erxue

Location: 1.2 cun lateral to the point Bixue. Indications: Deafness, tinnitus.

Kouxue

Location: On the mid-line of the planta, 1 cun anterior to the point Bixue.

Indications: Toothache, sore throat, tonsillitis.

Houxue

Location: On the mid-line of the planta, 0.6 cun anterior to the point Kouxue.

Indications: Fever, pharyngitis, tonsillitis, common cold.

Zaisheng

Location: On the mid-line of the planta, 0.6 cun anterior to the point Houxue.

Indications: Tumor of the intracranial part and spinal cord. Used for alleviating pain.

Xinxue

Location: On the mid-line of the planta, 0.5 cun anterior to the point Zaisheng.

Indications: Hypertension, heart failure, laryngitis, glossitis, insomnia, dreaminess.

Feixue

Location: 1 cun lateral and 0.1 cun posterior to the point Xinxue.

Indications: Cough with dyspnea, chest pain.

Anmian

Location: On the mid-line of the planta, 0.6 cun anterior to the point Xinxue.

Indications: Neurosis, schizophrenia, hysteria.

Weixue

Location: On the mid-line of the planta, 0.8 cun anterior to the point Anmian.

Indications: Stomachache, vomiting, indigestion.

Ganxue

Location: 1.2 cun medial to the point Weixue.

Indications: Chronic hepatitis, cholecystitis, ophthalmicdiseases, intercostal neuralgia.

Pixue

Location: 1.2 cun lateral to the point Weixue.

Indications: Indigestion, oliguria, hematopathy.

Danxue

Location: 0.3 cun posterior to the point Ganxue.

Indications: Cholecystitis, intercostal neuralgia.

Diaochangxue

Location: 1 cun ateral and 0.3 cun anterior to the point Weixue.

Indications: Abdominal pain with borborygmus.

Qianhouyinzhuxue

Location: Qianyinzhuxue is 0.4 cun anterior to the point Yongquan(KI1), Houyinzhuxue is 0.6 cun posterior to the point Yongquan(KI1).

Indications: Hypertension, schizophrenia, hysteria, high feverand coma.

Yongquanxue(KI1)

Indications: Hypertension, parietal headache, infantileconvulsion, shock, epilepsy.

Shenxue

Location: 1 cun lateral to Yongquan(KI1).

Indications: Hypertension, schizophrenia, acute lumbago, uroschesis.

Angen1

Location: 1 cun anterior to the point Ganxue.

Indications: Used for alleviating the pain due to tumor of thestomach, cardia and lower part of the esophagus.

Dachangxue

Location: The left Dangchangxue is 1.2 cun medial and 0.2 cunposterior to the point Houyinzhuxue, the right is 1.2 cun lateraland 0.2 cun posterior to the point Houyinzhuxue.

Indications: Abdominal pain, diarrhea, dysfunction of theintestine.

Gongsun(SP4)

Indications: Stomachache, vomiting, abdominal distention, indigestion.

Pangguangxue

Location: 1 cun anterior the point Yongquan(KI1).

Indications: uroschesis, enuresis, urinary incontinence.

Shengzhiqixue

Location: 0.3 cun anterior to the point Pangguangxue.

Indications: irregular menstruation, leukorrhagia, testitis, uroschesis.

Angen2

Location: 2 cun lateral and 0.1 cun anterior the pointPangguangxue.

Indications: Used for alleviating pain due to tumor of the organsin the lower abdomen and metastatic lymphoma.

Neilinqi

Location: On the planta, just below the point Zulinqi(GB41).

Indications: Migraine, pain in the hypochondria, ophthalmicdiseases, deafness, tinnitus, fever.

Neixiaxi
Location: On the planta, just below the point Xiaxi(GB43).

Indications: Migraine, pain in the hypochondria, ophthalmicdiseases, deafness, tinnitus, fever.

Lixiangu
Location: On the planta, just below the point Xiangu(ST43).

Indications: Acute stomachache, indigestion, schizophrenia.

Gangmenxue
Location: 0.6 cun anterior to the point Lixiangu.

Indications: Diarrhea, constipation.

Neitaichong
Location: On the planta, just below the point Taichong(LR3).

Indications: Testitis, hernia, dysfunctional uterine bleeding, irregular menstruation, leukorrhagia, dysmenorrhea, intercostalneuralgia, schizophrenia, hepatitis, hypertension, ophthalmicdiseases.

Lineiting
Location: On the planta, just below the point Neiting(ST3).

Indications: Infantile convulsion.

Duyin
Location: On the plantar side of the 2nd toe, at the center of the distal interphalangeal joint.

Indications: Hernia, dysmenorrhea, retention of placenta.

Muzhiliwenxue
Location: On the plantar side, at the center of the crossstriation of the 1st toe.

Indications: Testitis, pain due to hernia.

Aigen3
Location: 0.6 cun anterior to the point of Feixue of the medialside.

Indications: Used for alleviating pain due to tumor of theesophagus, lung, neck, and nasopharynx.

Qichuanxue
Location: At the toe tip.

Indications: Beriberi, numbness of the toes, thromboangiitisobliterans.

Zuxinxue
Location: At the midpoint of the mid-line of the plantar surface.

Indications: Neurosis, schizophrenia, hypertensive diseases.

Points on the Dorsum of Foot

Toutongdian
Location: On the dorsal surface of the foot, medial side of the 2nd, 3rd and 4th toes, and on the junction of the red and whiteskin.

Indications: Headache.

Biantao1
Location: On the metatarsophalangeal joint of the great toe, medial to the long extensor tendon of toe.

Indications: Tonsillitis, parotitis, eczema, urticaria.

Biantao2
Location: At the midpoint of the line connecting Taichong(LR3) and Xingjian(LR2).
Indications: Acute tonsillitis, parotitis.

Yaotongdian
Location: In the fossa anterolateral to capitulum of the first metatarsal bone.
Indications: Acute lumbar sprain, lumbago.

Zuogu2
Location: At the midpoint of the line connecting Zulinqi(GB41) and Diwului(GB43).
Indications: Sciatica.

Laozhen
Location: On the dorsum, 2 cun posterior to the junction of the red and white skin of the web connecting the 3rd and 4th toes.
Indications: Stiff neck.

Weichangdian
Location: On the dorsum, 3 cun posterior to the junction of the red and white skin of the web connecting the 2nd and 3rd toes.
Indications: Acute and chronic gastroenteritis, gastroduodenal ulcer.

Xintongdian
Location: 2.5 anterior to Jiexi(ST41).
Indications: Precordial pain, palpitation, asthma, common cold.

Yaotuidian
Location: In the fossa lateral to the point 0.5 cun anterior to Jiexi(ST41).
Indications: Lumbocrural pain, contraction of the lower extremities.

Points on the Medial Part of Foot

Xuanyundian
Location: In the fossa superior to the tuberosity of the navicular bone.
Indications: Dizziness, headache, hypertension, parotitis, acute tonsillitis.

Tongjing1
Location: 2 cun below the tip of the medial malleolus.
Indications: Dysmenorrhea, dysfunctional uterine bleeding, irregular menstruation.

Tongjing2
Location: In the fossa below the tuberosity of the navicular bone.
Indications: Dysmenorrhea, dysfunctional uterine bleeding, annexitis.

Dianxiandian
Location: At the midpoint of the line connecting Taibai(SP3) and Gongsun(SP4).
Indications: Epilepsy, hysteria, neurosis.

Bi
Location: 1 cun superior to Kunlun(BL60).

Indications: Sciatica, headache, abdominal pain.

New Points of Foot Acupuncture

1

Location: 1 cun superior to the midpoint of the posterior border of the planta.

Indications: Common cold, headache, rhinitis, maxillary sinusitis.

2

Location: 3 cun superior and 1 cun medial to the midpoint of the posterior border of the planta.

Indications: Prosopalgia.

3

Location: 3 cun superior to the midpoint of the posterior border of the planta.

Indications: Neurosis, hysteria, insomnia, hypotension, coma.

4

Location: 3 cun superior and 1 cun lateral to the midpoint of the posterior border of the planta.

Indications: Intercostal neuralgia, chest distress, chest pain.

5

Location: 4 cun superior and 1.5 cun lateral to the midpoint of the posterior border of the planta.

Indications: Sciatica, appendicitis, chest pain.

6

Location: 5 cun superior and 1 cun medial to the midpoint of the posterior border of the planta.

Indications: Dysentery, diarrhea, duodenal ulcer.

7

Location: 5 cun superior to the midpoint of the posterior border of the planta.

Indications: Asthma.

8

Location: 1 cun lateral to the point No. 8.

Indications: Neurosis, epilepsy.

9

Location: On the dorsum, 4 cun posterior to the junction of the red and white skin of the web connecting the great and 2nd toes.

Indications: Dysentery, diarrhea, inflammation of the uterus.

10

Location: 1 cun medial to Yongquan(KI1).

Indications: Gastroenteritis.

11

Location: 2 cun lateral to Yongquan(KI1).

Indications: Omalgia, urticaria.

12

Location: On the plantar surface, 1 cun posterior to the junction of the great and 2nd toes.

Indications: Toothache.

13

Location: On the plantar surface, 1 cun posterior to the midpoint of the cross striation of the little toe.
Indications: Toothache.

14

Location: At the midpoint of the cross striation of the little toe.
Indications: Enuresis, frequency of micturition.

15

Location: In the fossa lateral and 0.5 cun below the cross striation of ankle joint.
Indications: Lumbocrural pain, systremma.

16

Location: The same as the point Xuanyundian.
Indications: Hypertension, parotitis, acute tonsillitis.

17

Location: 2.5 cun below the midpoint of the cross striation of the ankle joint.
Indications: Angina pectoris, asthma, common cold.

18

Location: In the fossa anterolateral to the head of the first metatarsal bone.
Indications: Chest pain, chest distress, acute lumbar sprain.

19

Location: On the dorsum, 3 cun posterior to the junction of the 2nd and 3rd toes.
Indications: Headache, otitis media, acute and chronic gastroenteritis, gastroduodenal ulcer.

20

Location: On the dorsum, 2 cun posterior to the junction of the 3rd and 4th toes.
Indications: Stiff neck.

21

Location: On the dorsum, 0.5 cun posterior to the junction of the 4th and 5th toes.
Indications: Sciatica, parotitis, tonsillitis.

22

Location: On the dorsum, 1 cun posterior to the junction of the great and 2nd toes.
Indications: Acute tonsillitis, parotitis, hypertension.

23

Location: On the metatarsophalangeal joint medial to the long extensor tendon of the great toe.
Indications: Acute tonsillitis, parotitis, hypertension, prurigo nodularis, urticaria, eczema.

24

Location: On the junction of the red and white skin medial to the 2nd phalangeal joint of the 2nd toe.
Indications: Headache, otitis media

25

Location: On the junction of the red and white skin medial to the 2nd phalangeal joint of the 3rd toe.
Indications: Headache.

26

Location: On the junction of the red and white skin medial to the 2nd phalangeal joint of the 4th toe.
Indications: Headache, hypotension.

27

Location: At the midpoint of the line connecting Taibai(SP3) and Gongsun(SP4).
Indications: Epilepsy, hysteria, abdominal pain.

28

Location: In the fossa below and posterior to the tuberosity of the navicular bone.
Indications: Dysmenorrhea, dysfunctional uterine bleeding, adnexitis.

29

Location: 2 cun below the central point of the medial malleolus.
Indications: Dysfunctional uterine bleeding, trachitis, asthma.

30

Location: 1.5 cun posterior and superior to the external malleolus.
Indications: Sciatica, lumbago, headache.

Chapter Fourteen
Points of Wrist and Ankle Acupuncture

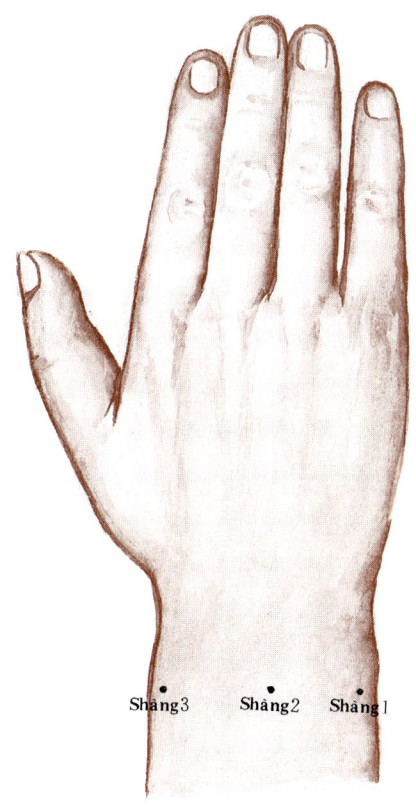
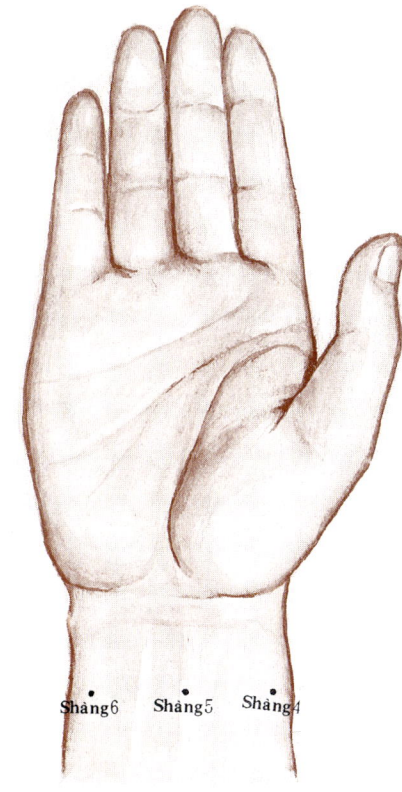
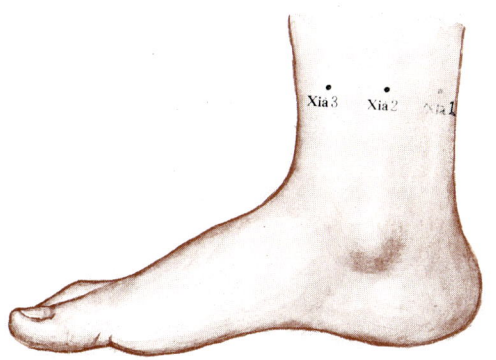
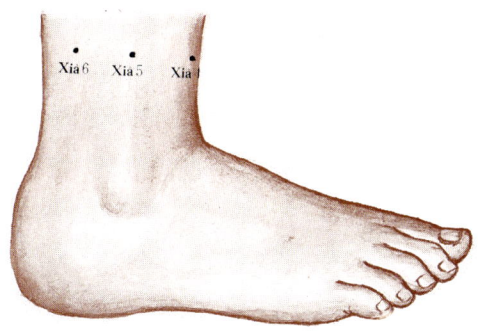

Fig. 40

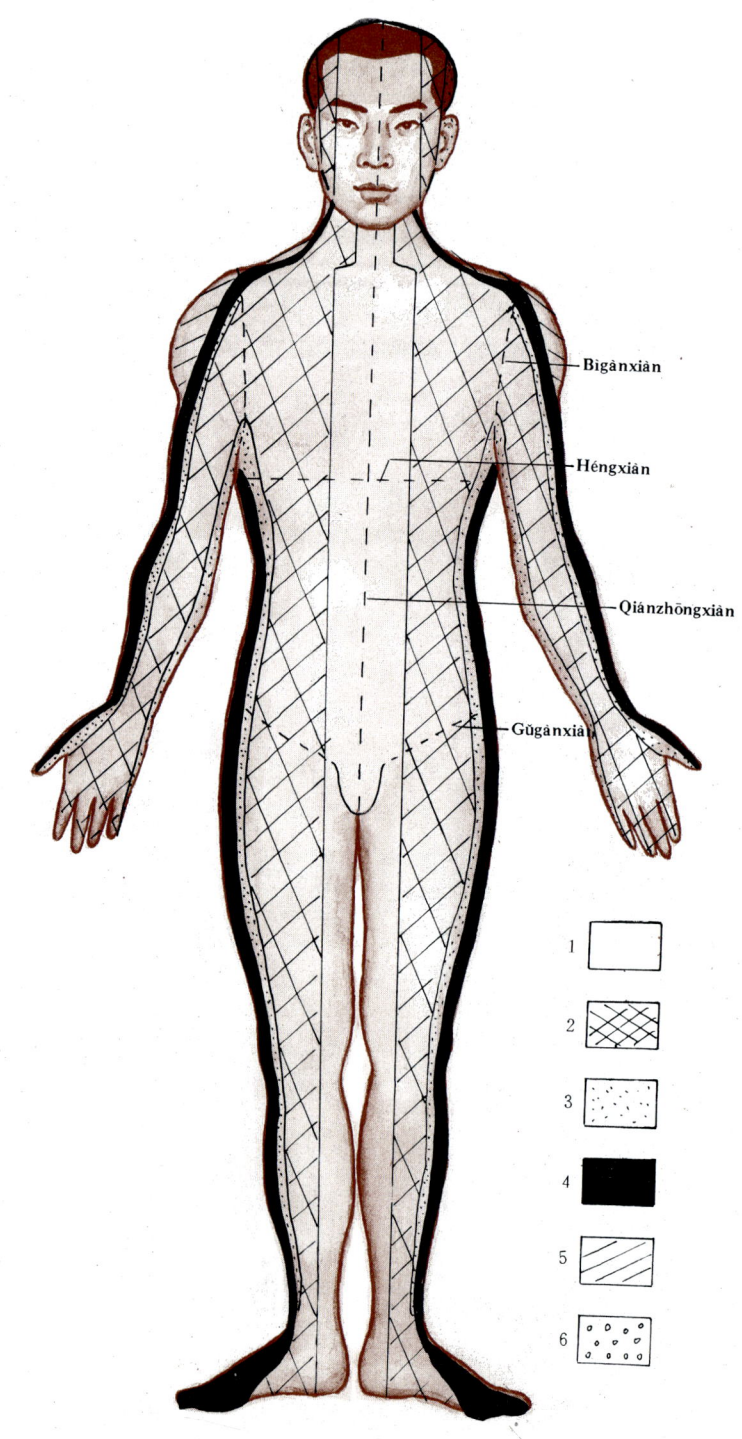

Fig. 41

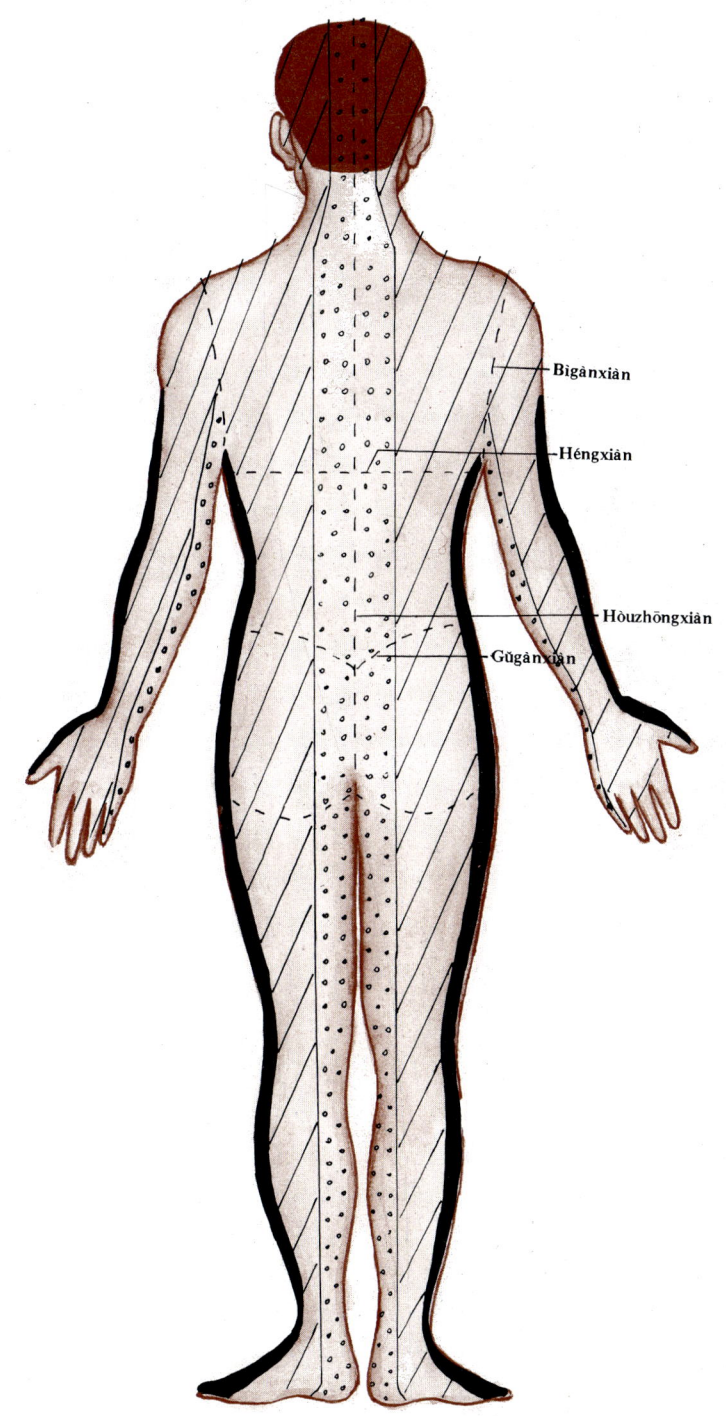

Fig. 42

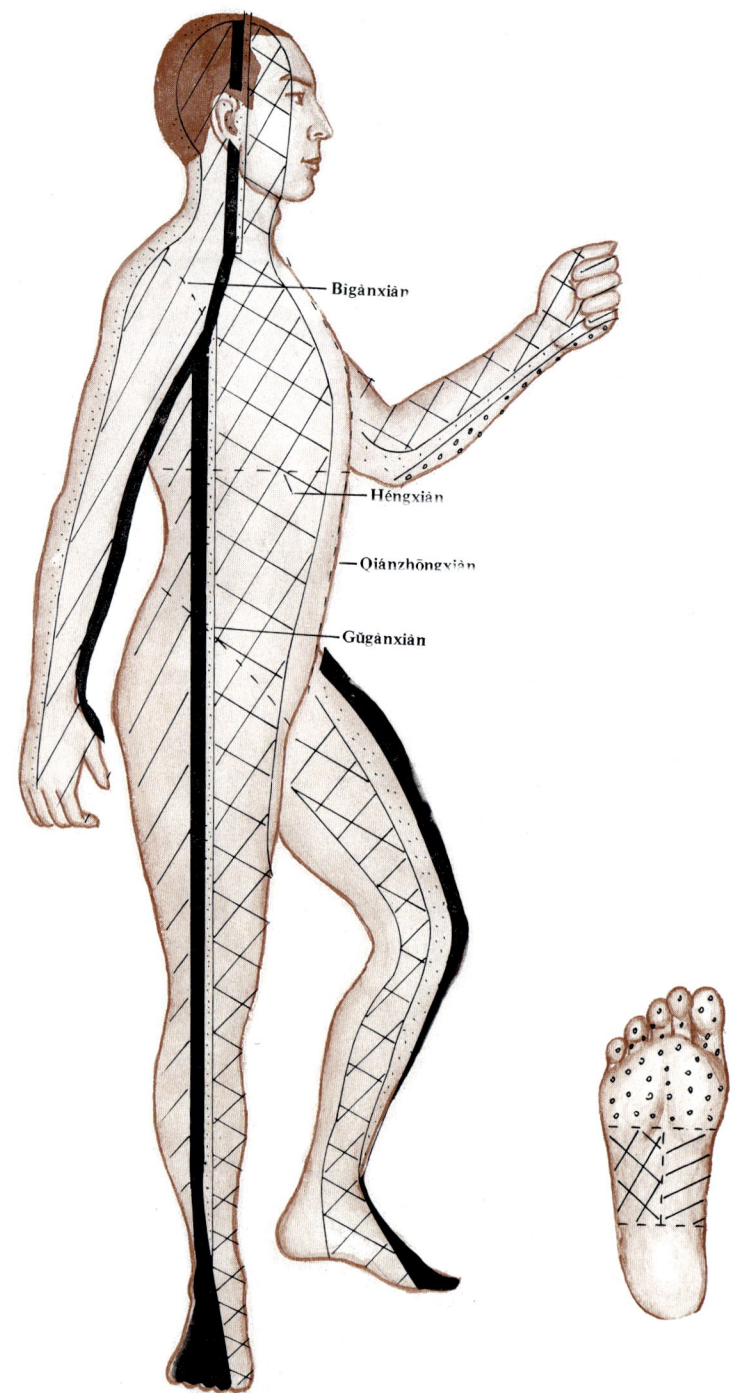

Fig. 43

Points on the Wrist

There are six points on a horizontal ring 2 fingers breadths superior to cross striation of the wrist, which are respectively named Shang1, 2, 3, 4, 5, and 6.

Shang1

Location: In the fossa between the ulna and ulnar flexor tendon of the wrist.

Indications: Headache in the forehead, ophthalmic diseases, rhinopathy, prosopalgia, swelling of the face, toothache, dizziness, sore throat, trachitis, stomachache, heart diseases, hypertension, night sweat, chill, insomnia, hysteria.

Shang2

Location: On the palmar surface of the wrist, just between tendon palmaris longus and tendon flexor carpi radialis.

Indications: Headache in the forehead, toothache, swelling of the mandible, chest distress, chest pain, asthma, pain in the palm, numbness of the finger tip.

Shang3

Location: On the radial side of arteria radialis, medial border of the radius.

Indications: hypertension, chest pain

Shang4

Location: On the lateral border of the radius.

Indications: Headache in the vertex, otopathy, dysfunction of temporal mandibular joint, scapulohumeral periarthritis, chestpain.

Shang5

Location: On the dorsal carpal surface, between radius and ulna.

Indications: Headache in the posterior temporal portion, paresthesia or dyscinesia of the upper limbs, pain in the elbow, carpal and interphalangeal articulations of hand.

Shang6

Location: On the lateral side of the ulna, on the dorsal carpal surface.

Indications: headache in the occiput, pain in the neck and cervical vertebrae, rachialgia.

Points on the Ankle

There are six points on a horizontal ring 3 fingers breadths superior to the upper border of the ankle, which are respectively named Xia1, 2, 3, 4, 5, and 6.

Xia1

Location: On the medial border of Achilles tendon.

Indications: Distention of the gastric region, periumbilical pain, dysmenorrhea, leukorrhagia, pruritus vulvae, enuresis, painful heels

Xia2

Location: On the medial surface of the tibia, near the posterior border.

Indications: Hepatalgia, pain in the lateral portion of the abdomen, irritable colon.

Xia3

Location: 1 cm medial and posterior to the anterior border of the tibia.

Indications: Gonalgia in the medial portion

Xia4

Location: Just between the anterior border of the tibia and that of the fibula.

Indications: Aching pain in the musculus quadriceps femoris, gonalgia, paresthesia or dyscinesia of the lower limbs, pain in the phalangeal joint.

Xia5

Location: On the lateral surface of the leg, near the posterior border of the tibia.

Indications: Pain in the hip joint, sprain of ankle.

Xia6

Location: On the lateral border of Achilles tendon.

Indications: Acute lumbar sprain, lumbar muscle strain, pain in the sacro-iliac joint, sciatica, systremma.

Chapter Fifteen
Points of Meridians and Collaterals-Point Area and Belt Acupuncture

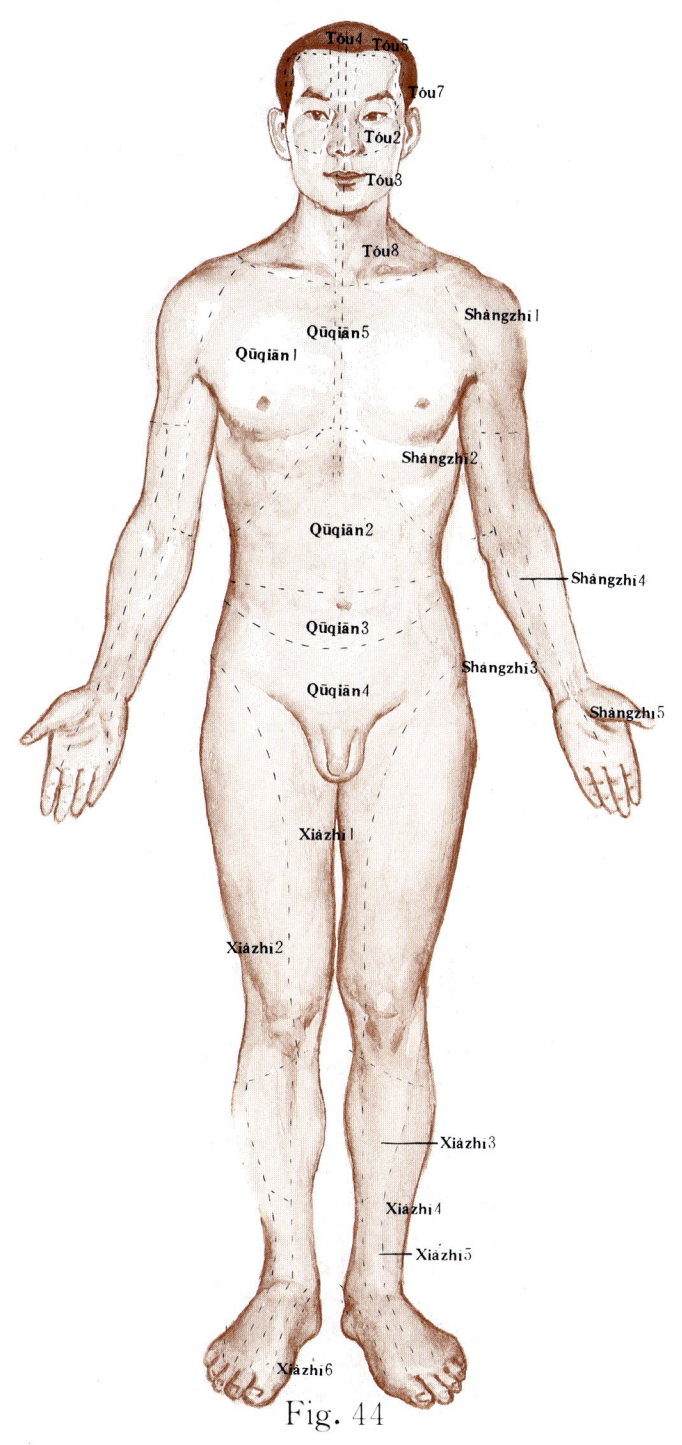

Fig. 44

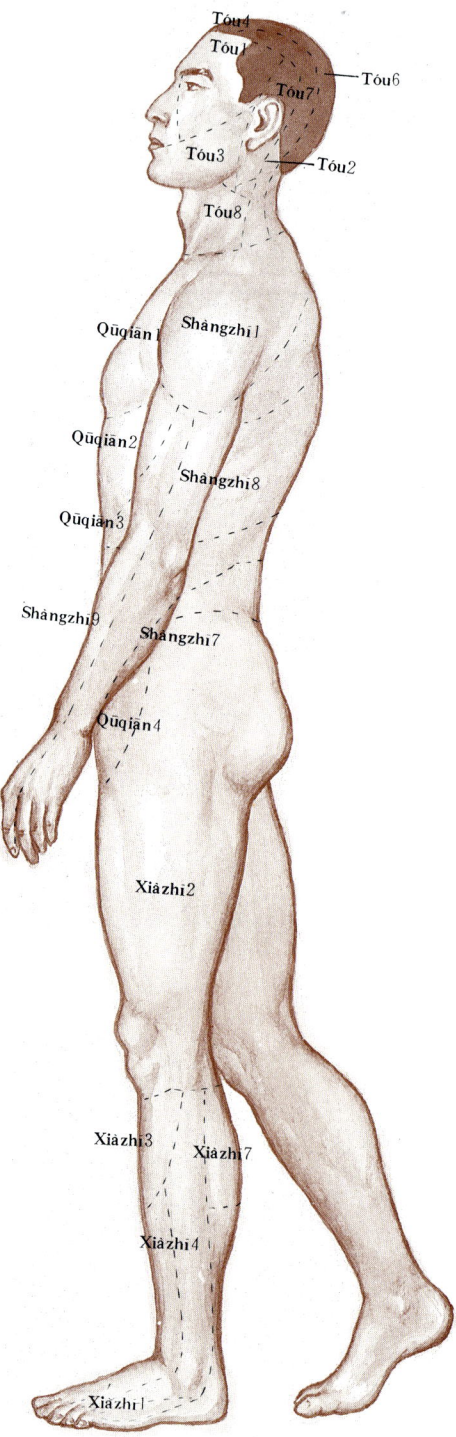

Fig. 45

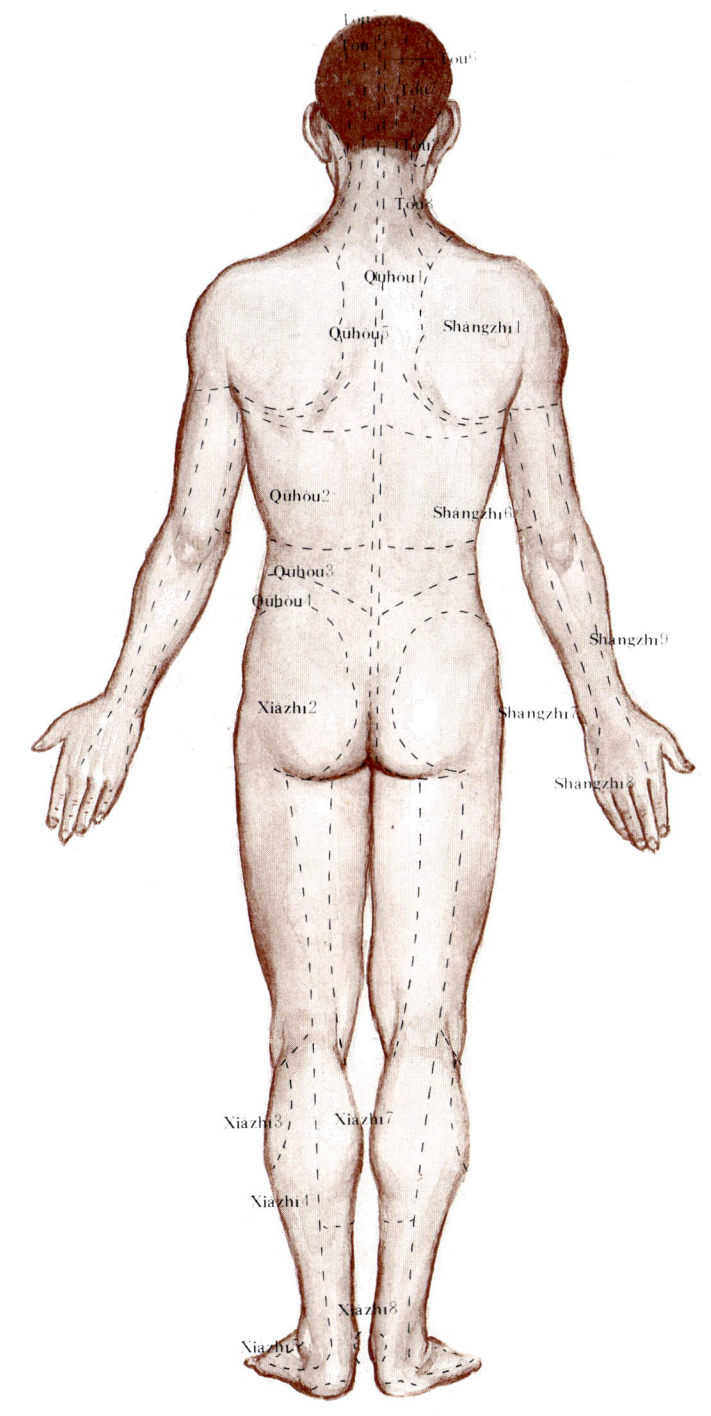

Fig. 46

Tou1

Indications: Ophthalmic disorders, headache in the peripheralportion.

Tou2

Indications: Otopathy, headache in the peripheral portion.

Tou3

Indications: Disorders affected the mouth, teeth, mandible andcheek, localized headache.

Tou4

Indications: rhinopathy.

Tou5

Indications: Encephalopathy, neuropathy, mental diseases.

Tou6

Indications: Encephalopathy, neuropathy, Ophthalmic disorders,migraine. Also effective for rhinopathy and otopathy.

Tou7

Indications: Migraine, toothache. Tou8

Indications: Disorders affecting the tongue, pharynx, larynx, andneck.

Quqian1

Indications: Disorders distributed to the chest and hypochondria,especially to the heart and lung.

Quqian2

Indications: Gastrointestinal disorders, hepatopathy, psychosis.

Quqian3

Indications: Gastrointestinal disorders, diseases of urogenitalsystem.

Quqian4

Indications: Diseases of urogenital system, intestinal diseases.

Quqian5

Indications: Psychosis, disorders distributed to the head andface.

Quhou1

Indications: Fever, disorders distributed to the heart, lung, andstomach, psychosis.

Quhou2

Indications: Hepatic and gastrointestinal disorders.

Quhou3

Indications: Disorders distributed to the liver, intestine,kidney and genitals, lumbago, hemorrhoid.

Quhou4

Indications: Disorders of urogenital system, lumbago, hemorrhoid.

Quhou5

Indications: Psychosis, Disorder of nervous system.

Shangzhi1

Indications: Disorders distributed to the nape, shoulder,scapular region, arm and chest, psychosis.

Shangzhi2

Indications: Disorders distributed to the shoulder, arm, chestand hypochondrium, psychosis, ophthalmic disorders.

Shangzhi3

Indications: Heart disorders.

Shangzhi4

Indications: heart and gastric disorders, psychosis, fever.

Shangzhi5

Indications: Disorders distributed to the neck, pharynx and larynx, lung disorders, psychosis.

Shangzhi6

Indications: Disorders distributed to the neck, cheek, teeth and ear, psychosis, pain in the scapula.

Shangzhi7

Indications: Disorders distributed to the head, ear, nose, nape, larynx and pharynx, fever, psychosis.

Shangzhi8

Indications: Disorders distributed to the head, ear, eye, larynx and pharynx, fever, psychosis.

Shangzhi9

Indications: Disorders distributed to the head, ear, eye, larynx and pharynx, nape and chest, fever, intestinal disorders.

Xiazhi1

Indications: Disorders of urogenital system, gastrointestinal disorders, disorders distributed to the larynx and pharynx.

Xiazhi2

Indications: Lumbocrural pain, disorders distributed to the lower extremities.

Xiazhi3

Indications: Gastrointestinal disorders, psychosis.

Xiazhi4

Indications: Disorders distributed to the head, ear, eye, larynx and pharynx, chest and hypochondrium, fever.

Xiazhi5

Indications: Disorders distributed to the head, eye, nose, teeth, shoulder, gastrointestinal disorders, psychosis.

Xiazhi6

Indications: Gastrointestinal disorders, hemorrhoid, psychosis, fever.

Xiazhi7

Indications: Lumbago, psychosis, disorders of the urinary system.

Xiazhi8

Indications: Disorders distributed to the head, eye, nose and neck, psychosis, fever, disorders of urogenital system.

Chapter Sixteen
Points in Infantile Massage

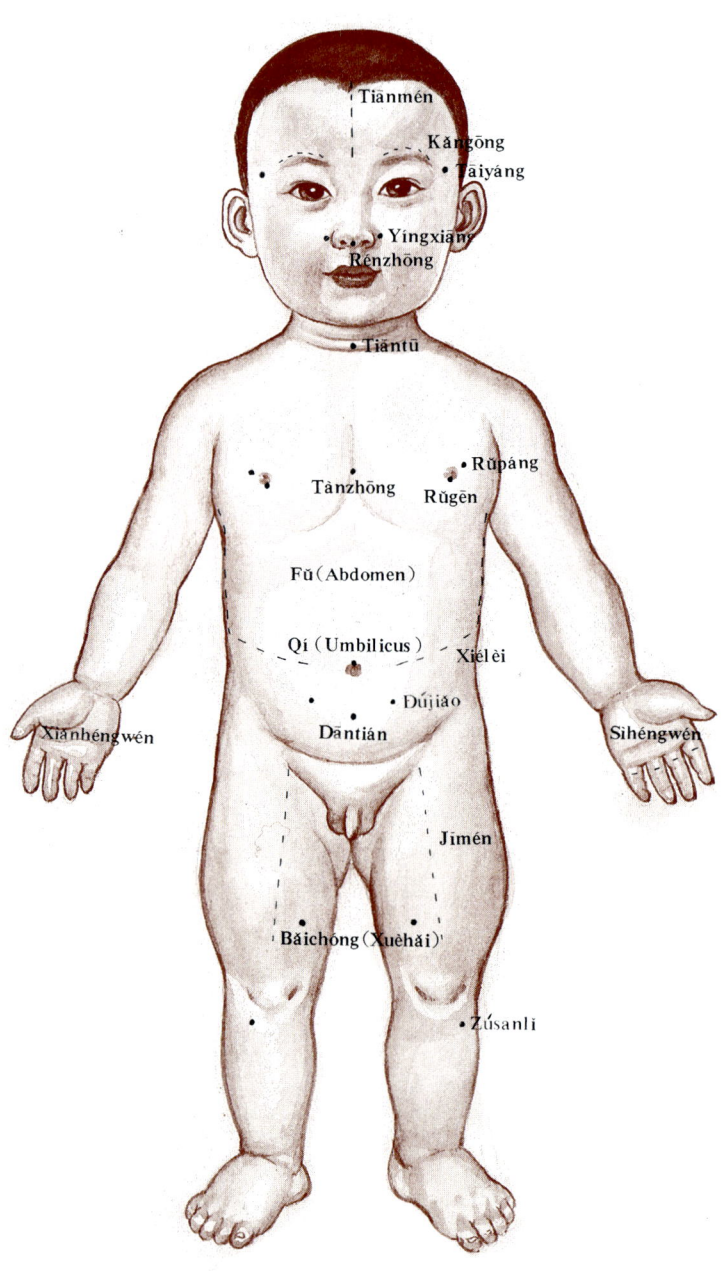

Fig. 47

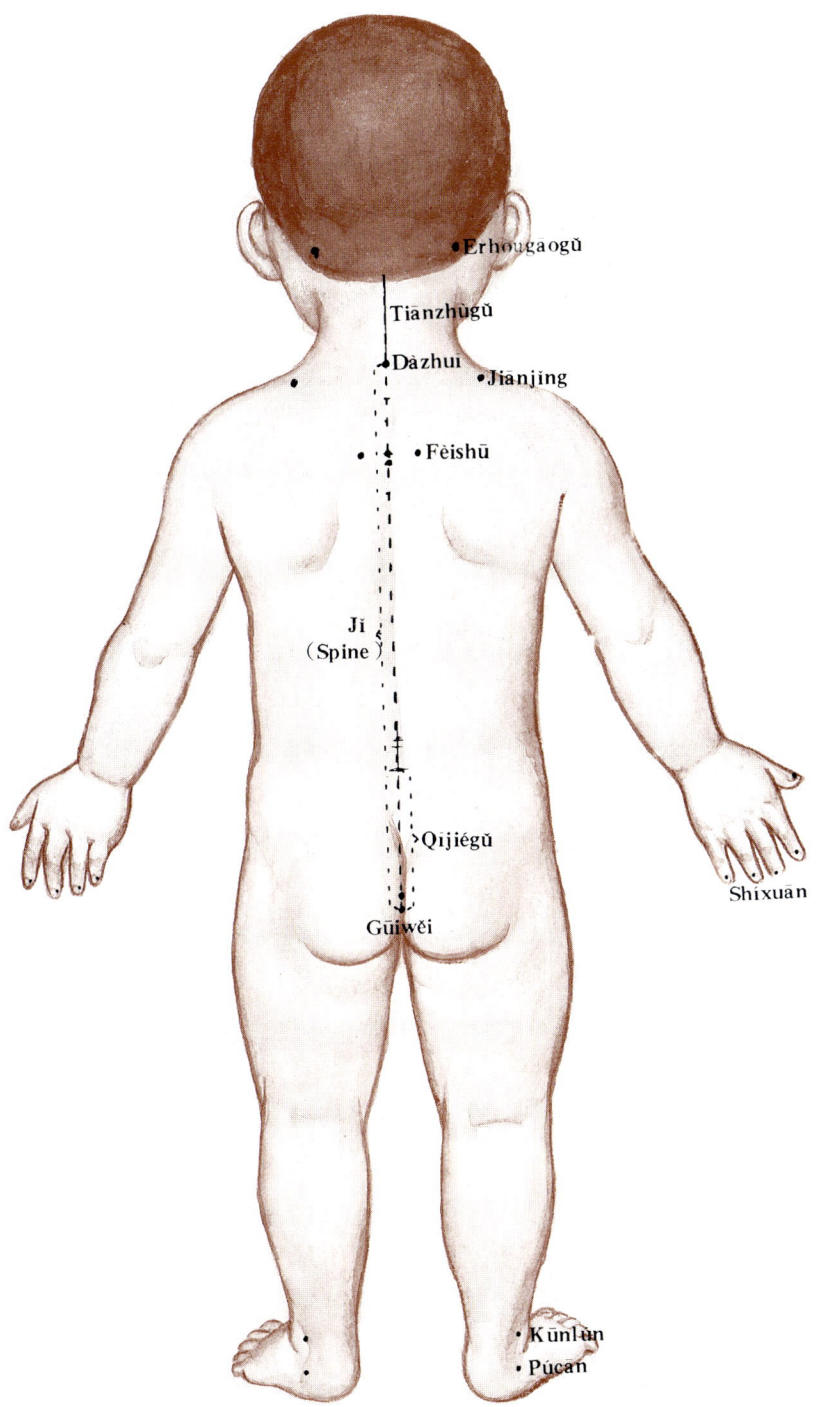

Fig. 48

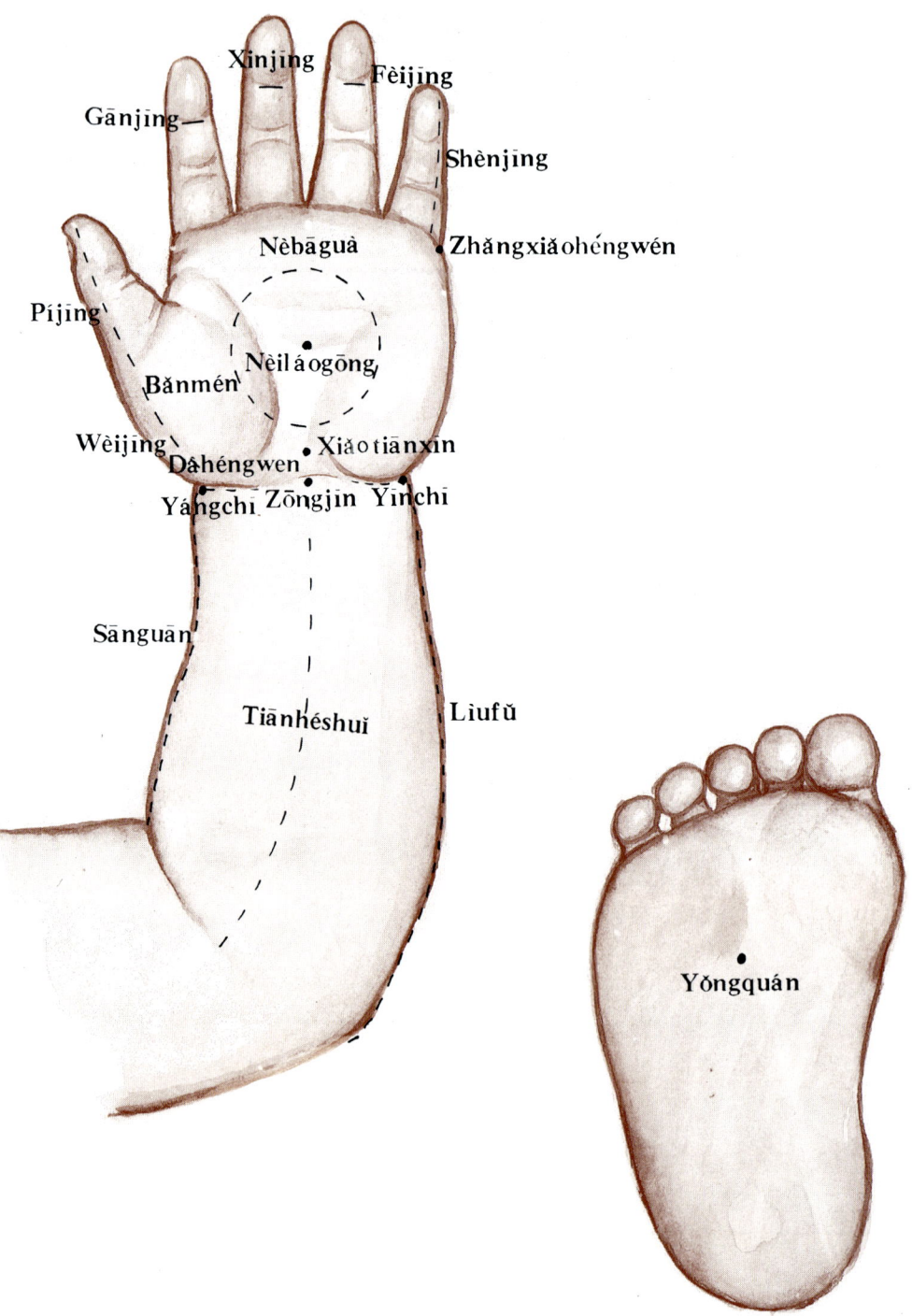

Fig. 49

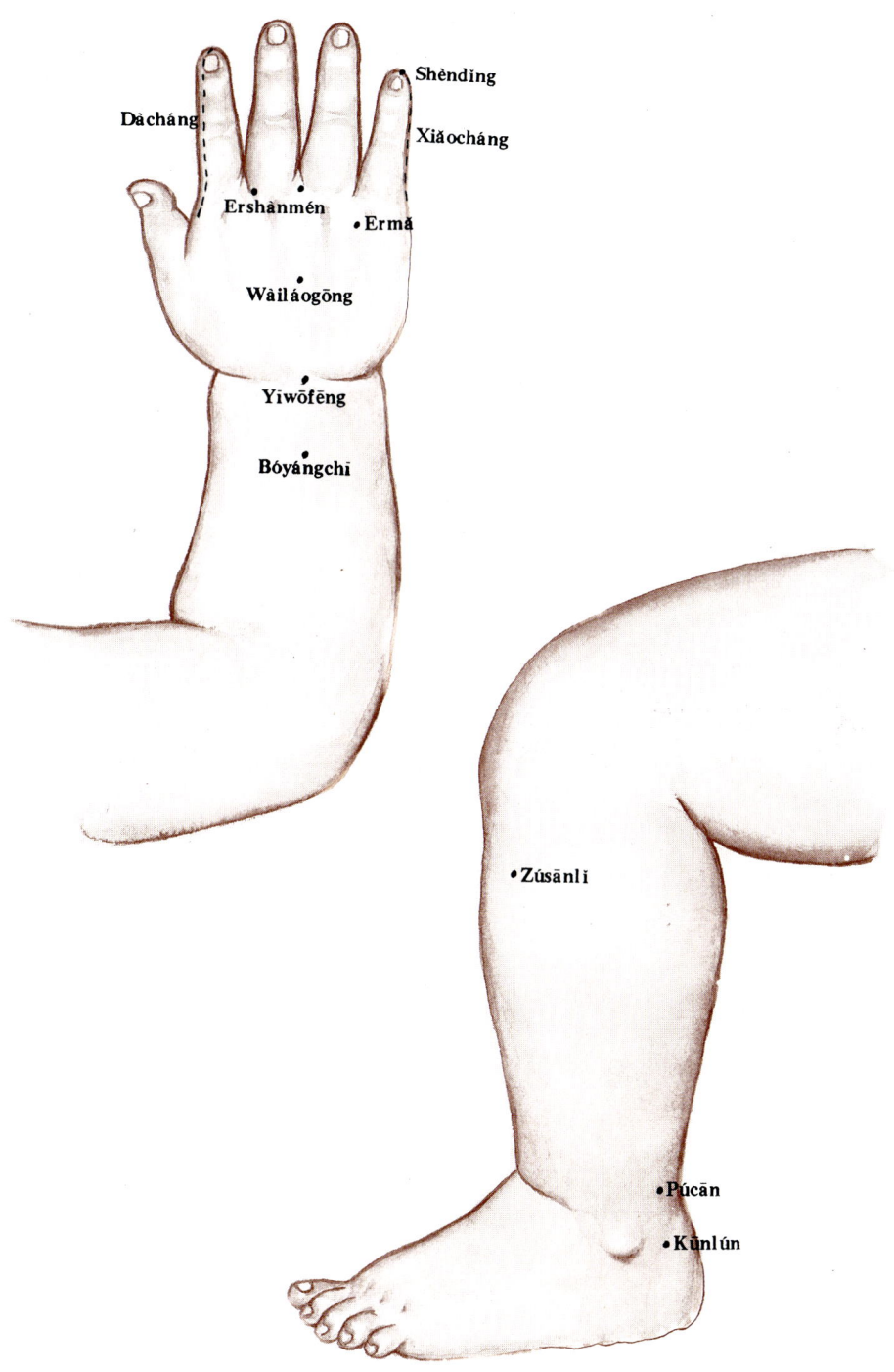

Fig. 50

1. Points on the Head and Face

Tianmen

Location: The part above the line between the eyebrows up to the anterior hair line.

Indications: Fever, headache, cold with anhidrosis or with obstructed sweating, listlessness, vigilance and restlessness.

Kangong

Location: Along the eyebrow from the beginning to the end.

Indications: Fever due to exogenous evils, headache, dizziness, conjunctival congestion with pain, infantile convulsion.

Taiyang(EX-HN5)

Location: In the depression about 1.0 cun posterior to the midpoint between the lateral ends of the eyebrows and the outer canthus.

Indications: Cold, fever, headache, infantile convulsion, conjunctival congestion with pain.

Erhougaogu

Location: In the depression inferior to postauditory process and superior to retroauricular hairline.

Indications: Cold due to pathogenic wind, headache, infantile convulsion, restlessness, dizziness, redness, swelling and pain of the eye.

Renzhong(DU26)

Location: At the junction of the superior 1/3 and middle 2/3 of the philtrum.

Indications: Infantile convulsion, syncope, tic.

Yingxiang(LI20)

Location: 0.5 cun lateral to the midpoint of the lateral border of ala nasi, in the nasolabial groove.

Indication: Cold due to pathogenic wind, stuffed running nose, chronic rhinitis.

Tianzhugu

Location: The straight line from the middle of the hairline to Dazhui(DU14).

Indications: Vomiting, nausea, stiffness of the neck, fever, sore throat, infantile convulsion.

2. Points on the Chest and Abdomen

Tiantu(RN22)

Location: At the center of the suprasternal fossa.

Indications: Stuffiness in the chest, cough with dyspnea, accumulation of phlegm with rapid breathing, nausea, vomiting, sore throat.

Danzhong(RN17)

Location: On the anterior midline at the level with the fourth intercostal space, midpoint between the two nipples.

Indications: Stuffiness in the chest, rale, cough, dyspnea, vomiting, nausea, hiccup, etc.

Rugen(RN18)

Location: 0.2 cun below the breast.

Indications: Stuffiness in the chest, chest pain, cough, dyspnea.

Rupang

Location: 0.2 cun lateral to the breast.

Indications: Stuffiness in the chest, cough, rale, vomiting.

Xielei(Hypochondrium)

Location: From the two hypochondria under the armpits to Tianshu(ST25).

Indications: Stuffiness in the chest, hypochondriac pain, abdominal distention, phlegm-dyspnea, rapid breathing, infantile malnutrition, hepatosplenomegaly.

Fu

Location: On the abdomen.

Indications: Abdominal pain, abdominal distention, indigestion, nausea, vomiting, food retention in stomach, and anorexia, constipation.

Umbilicus(Shenque, RN8)

Location: In the center of the umbilicus.

Indications: Abdominal distention, abdominal pain, dyspepsia, constipation, borborygmus, vomiting and diarrhea.

Dantian

Location: On the lower abdomen, between 2 and 3 cun under the umbilicus.

Indications: Pain in the lower abdomen, diarrhea, enuresis, prolapse of rectum, hernia, uroschesis, scanty dark urine, weakness.

Dujiao

Location: Lateral to the umbilicus, on the strong tendons of both sides of the abdomen.

Indications: Abdominal pain, diarrhea, abdominal distention, dysentery, constipation.

3. Points on the Lumbodorsal Area

Jianjing(GB21)

Location: Midway between Dazhui(DU14) and the acromion.

Indications: Cold, infantile convulsion, raising disorder of the upper limbs.

Dazhui(DU14)

Location: Below the spinous process of the 7th cervical vertebra.

Indications: Cold, fever, stiffness of neck, cough, whooping cough.

Feishu(BL13)

Location: 1.5 cun lateral to the lower borer of the spinous process of the 3rd thoracic vertebra.

Indications: Cough, asthma, rale, stuffiness and pain in the chest, fever.

Ji(Spine)

Location: The straight line between Dazhui(DU14) and Changqiang(DU1).

Indications: Cold, fever, constipation, vomiting and acute infantile convulsion, malnutrition, diarrhea, abdominal pain, chronic infantile convulsion, anorexia, muscular emaciation.

Qijiegu

Location: The line from the fourth lumbar vertebra to caudal vertebra.

Indications: Diarrhea of asthenia-cold type, persistent dysentery, enuresis, prolapse of rectum, constipation due to heat in the bowel, dysentery, abdominal distention.

Guiwei
Location: At the end of caudal vertebra.

Indications: Diarrhea, dysentery, constipation, prolapse of rectum, enuresis.

4. Points on the Upper Limbs

Pijing
Location: On the red-white border of the radial surface of the thumbs, the straight line from the finger tip to the end.

Indications: Debility, anorexia, emaciation of muscle, lassitude and indigestion, jaundice, dampness-phlegm syndrome, hematochezia, nausea, vomiting, diarrhea, dysentery, constipation, fullness in the stomach, acid regurgitation, anorexia, diarrhea, vomiting.

Ganjing
Location: At the end part of the index finger of the palm area.

Indications: Infantile convulsion, conjunctival congestion, restlessness, dysphoria with feverish sensation in the chest, palms and soles, bitter taste, dry throat, dizziness, headache, tinnitus, etc.

Xinjing
Location: At the end part of the middle finger on palm surface.

Indications: Pyrexia with delirium, dysphoria with feverish sensation in the chest, palms and soles, oral ulceration, difficulty and dark urine, frightening with restlessness, sweating due to deficiency of heart blood, listlessness, restlessness, sleeping with eyes open.

Feijing
Location: At palm surface of the end of the ring finger.

Indications: Cold, fever, cough, dyspnea, rale, stuffiness in the chest, cough due to insufficiency of lung-qi, shortness of breath, pale face, spontaneous perspiration, chillness and prolapse of rectum.

Shenjing
Location: From the tip of little finger to the root of palm, on the palm aspect of the little finger, slightly towards ulna.

Indications: Congenital defect, weakness due to chronic disease, chronic diarrhea due to kidney deficiency, polyuria, enuresis, sweating due to debility, dyspnea, dark urine

Dachang
Location: The edge of the radial surface of the index finger, or the straight line from the tip of the finger to the part which is between the thumb and the index finger.

Indications: Diarrhea of asthenia-cold type, prolapse of rectum, fever, abdominal pain, dysentery, indigestion and diarrhea due to damp-heat, bitter taste and dry throat, constipation, pain in the chest and hypochondrium, red and swollen anus.

Xiaochang
Location: On the ulnar edge of the little finger, the straight way from the tip of little finger to the end.

Indications: Scanty dark urine, anuresis, watery diarrhea, hectic fever in the afternoon, polyuria, enuresis.

Shending
Location: On the tip of the little finger.

Indications: Spontaneous perspiration, night sweat, infantile metopism.

Sihengwen
Location: On the cross-striation area of the first finger joint of the index, middle, ring, and little fingers on the palm.

Indications: Infantile malnutrition, abdominal distention and pain, derangement of qi and blood, indigestion, infantile convulsion, dyspnea, cracked lips, infantile malnutrition.

Xiaohengwen
Location: At the cross-striation area of metacarpophalangeal articulation of the index, middle, ring and little fingers on the palm aspect.

Indications: Cracked lips, aphthae, fever, restlessness, abdominal flatulence.

Zhangxiaohengwen
Location: At the edge of ulnar palm print, the end of the little finger on the palm aspect.

Indications: Dyspnea and cough due to heat and phlegm, aphthae, slobbering, pneumonia, whooping cough.

Weijing
Location: On the red-white border of the radial surface of the major thenar eminence.

Indications: Nausea, vomiting, hiccup, eructation, excessive thirst and desire for food, hematemesis and nosebleeding.

Banmen
Location: On the flat area of the major thenar eminence of palm.

Indications: Dyspepsia, abdominal flatulence, anorexia, vomiting, diarrhea, dyspnea, eructation.

Neilaogong
Location: In the center of the palm at the midpoint between the bent middle and ring finger.

Indications: Fever, excessive thirst, aphthae, erosion of gum, asthenia-type restlessness with heat in the interior.

Neibagua
Location: On palm surface. Taking the center of the palm as the center of a circle and 2/3 from the center of the circle to the cross striation of the middle finger as the radius, draw a circle. The circle is Neibagua.

Indications: Cough with phlegm-dyspnea, stuffiness in the chest with anorexia, abdominal distention, vomiting, diarrhea, loss of appetite.

Xiaotianxin
Location: In the depression of the intersection point of major thenar eminence and minor thenar eminence at the root of palm.

Indications: Conjunctival congestion with pain, aphthae, convulsion with restlessness, scanty, dark urine, scleroderma neonatorum, jaundice, enuresis, edema, sore furuncle, measles with incomplete eruption, convulsion, night cry, restlessness, strabismus, somnambulism.

Zongjin
Location: On the middle of the cross striation, at the palm surface of the wrist.

Indications: Infantile convulsion, spasm, night cry, aphthae, hectic fever, toothache, and borborygmus with vomiting and diarrhea.

Dahengwen
Location: At the cross striation of the wrist, on the palmar aspect. Yangchi is near the thumb. Yinchi is near the

little finger.

Indications: Alternating episodes of chills and fever, diarrhea, vomiting, dysentery, abdominal distention, indigestion, persistent fever, restlessness, infantile convulsion, spasm and abundant expectoration.

Shixuan (EX-UE11)

Location: On the tips of the ten fingers, about 0.1 cun distal to the nails.

Indications: Acute fever with convulsion, spasm, heat syndromes of the heart, restlessness and trance.

Ershanmen

Location: In the depression on both sides of the caput of the third ossa metacarpi on the dorsum of the hand.

Indications: Convulsion, fever with anhidrosis, cold, phlegm-dyspnea, difficult respiration, acute convulsion, facial hemiparalysis.

Erma

Location: In the depression of the metacarpophalangeal articulations of the ring and little finger on the dorsum of the hand.

Indications: Fever of deficiency type and cough with dyspnea, scanty dark urine and dribbling urination, abdominal pain, weakness, stranguria, prolapse of rectum, enuresis, indigestion, toothache, teeth-grinding while sleeping, dyspnea.

Wailaogong

Location: On the dorsum of hand, opposite to Neilaogong.

Indications: Common cold of wind-cold type, abdominal pain, abdominal distention, borborygmus, diarrhea, dysentery, prolapse of rectum, enuresis, cough, dyspnea, hernia.

Yiwofeng

Location: In the depression in the middle of the transverse crease of the wrist on the dorsum of hand.

Indications: Invasion by wine, cold, abdominal pain, borborygmus, arthralgia and acute or chronic convulsion.

Boyangchi

Location: 3 cun posterior to Yiwofeng, between the ulna and radius on the dorsal aspect of the forearm.

Indications: Cold, headache, constipation, dark urine.

Sanguan

Location: The straight way from the transverse crease of the wrist to the transverse crease of the elbow, on the radial aspect of the forearm.

Indications: All kinds of cold of insufficiency type, weakness after illness, insufficiency of yang and cold extremities, myasthenia of limbs, abdominal pain, diarrhea, macular eruption and miliaria alba, measles with incomplete appearance of rashes, infantile acroparalysis.

Liufu

Location: At the ulnar part of the forearm, the straight way from the transverse crease of the elbow to the wrist.

Indications: All kinds of sthenic-heat syndrome such as high fever, restlessness, thirst and desire for cold water, infantile convulsion, thrush, swollen and rigid tongue, double tongue, sore throat, mumps, pyogenic infections and dysentery of heat type.

Tianheshui

Location: The straight way from the transverse crease of wrist to the elbow, in the middle of medial aspect of the forearm.

Indications: All kinds of heat syndrome.

5. Points on the Lower Limbs

Jimen
Location: In the medial aspect of thighs, the straight way from the superior border of the knee to the groin.
Indications: Scanty dark urine, anuresis, watery diarrhea.

Baichong
Location: 2 cun directly above the medial border of the patella.
Indications: Convulsion, coma, unconsciousness, paralysis of lower limbs, arthralgia-syndrome.

Zusanli(ST36)
Location: 3 cun below Oubi (ST35), one finger-breadth from the anterior crest of the tibia.
Indications: Abdominal distention, abdominal pain, diarrhea, vomiting, flaccidity of lower limbs.

Pucan(BL61)
Location: 2 cun directly below Kunlun (BL60).
Indications: Infantile convulsion, spasm, faint, sprain of lateral malleolus.

Yongquan(KI1)
Location: At the junction between anterior 1/3 and posterior 2/3 of the sole, in the depression when the foot is in plantar flexion.
Indications: Dysphoria with feverish sensation in the chest, palms and soles, restlessness at night, fever, vomiting, diarrhea.

(京)新登字 207 号

图书在版编目(CIP)数据

ATLAS COLLECTION OF ACUPUNCTURE & MASSAGE＝中国针灸推拿图谱大全：英文/赵昕主编；李国华译.-北京：北京科学技术出版社，1996.1
ISBN 7-5304-1835-1
Ⅰ.A… Ⅱ.①赵… ②李… Ⅲ.①针灸疗法-中国-图谱 ②按摩疗法(中医)-图谱 Ⅳ.R245-64
中国版本图书馆 CIP 数据核字（96）第 00042 号

中国针灸推拿图谱大全

主编 赵　昕

翻译　李国华

绘图　王东升

北京科学技术出版社出版
（中国北京西直门南大街 16 号）
邮政编码　100035
北京大兴沙窝店印刷厂印刷
中国国际图书贸易总公司发行
（中国北京车公庄西路 35 号）
北京邮政信箱第 399 号　邮政编码 100044
787×1092 毫米　16 开本　英文版
1996 年 1 月第一版　1996 年 1 月第一次印刷
ISBN 7-5304-1835-1/R・352

06860
14-E-2991 P